THE BODY SPEAKS

THE BODY SPEAKS

Therapeutic Dialogues for
Mind-Body Problems

JAMES L. GRIFFITH
MELISSA ELLIOTT GRIFFITH

BasicBooks
A Division of HarperCollinsPublishers

Designed by Ellen Levine

Library of Congress Cataloging-in-Publication Data

Griffith, James L., 1950-
    The body speaks : therapeutic dialogues for mind-body problems / James
L. Griffith, Melissa Elliott Griffith.
            p.   cm.
    Includes bibliographical references and index.
    ISBN 0-465-00716-3
    1. Medicine, Psychosomatic. 2. Mind and body therapies.
I. Griffith, Melissa Elliott, 1952- . II. Title.
RC49.G645 1994
616.08—dc20   93-34330
                                                                CIP

94 95 96 97 ❖/HC 9 8 7 6 5 4 3 2 1

For our children,
Marianna Louise Griffith
and Van Elliott Griffith,
who have made our lives more delightful
than we ever could have imagined

Contents

Acknowledgments

TO BE MARRIED to one's coauthor has been a growing, challenging experience for each of us. Surely there can be no freedom to develop one's work and ideas like the freedom that comes from being with a partner whose love and respect are present whether one is creative and successful or not.

For the gift of this marriage and the freedom it makes possible, we thank our parents, Louise and Lamont Griffith and Van and Helen Elliott.

For the appreciation of this partnership and our differences that made creativity possible, we thank our family therapy colleagues, teachers, and trainees. We feel deep gratitude for Harry Goolishian, who renewed in us an excitement about language and helped us to work with persons in therapy in a way that fosters respect for them and for ourselves. Through Harry we met Tom Andersen, Anna Margrete-Flam, Magnus Hald, and their colleagues from northern Norway, who inspired us to reflect on our clinical practices and to let go of therapeutic agendas that obstructed our being in language with others. These friendships began a collaboration that took us to Norway and our Norwegian colleagues to Mississippi on numerous occasions. More than any other single clinician, our clinical work has been shaped by our conversations and friendship with Tom Andersen. Over breakfast in New Orleans several years ago, Tom shared an idea that eventually gave this book its direction—we should not speak about language as having digital and analogical aspects but rather digital and physiological aspects.

Many creative ideas and fruitful professional relationships came through the generosity of our friend and colleague Sallyann Roth, who shared with us her considerable knowledge and skills in systemic therapy, then made certain to include us in conversations with therapists whose work she recognized as being on the cutting edge of the field. It was, in fact, at her urging that we invited Michael and Cheryl White from Australia to Mississippi, a visit that expanded our vision beyond the processes of nuclear families to the wider cultural and social practices that shape families. We learned from Michael and Cheryl and, later, David Epston from New Zealand how to deconstruct oppressive social practices and to reconstruct with persons the guiding narratives that they preferred to organize their lives. In the work of other New Zealand friends, Charles Waldegrave, Kiwi Tamasese, and Betsan Martin at the Anglican Family Centre in Lower Hutte, we saw a way to live out the inseparable connection of family therapy and social justice. Our colleagues Gene Combs and Jill Freedman encouraged us with their work and with their own partnership. So many other colleagues, at home and far away, have discussed and agreed and disagreed but have been willing to stay in the conversation, helping us to change and to grow.

Those who have helped us most to change and grow, of course, are those persons who were willing to come as patients and families. They often reflected on a session with us and showed us what was useful, as well as what we might have done differently, shaping how we decided to work in the future and what we decided to write about here.

For each of us there has been a special friend and clinician, who from the earliest days of training until the present has encouraged each of us to dream and has been a constant help in giving life to these dreams. For Melissa, this is Martha Jurchak. For James, this is Lois Slovik.

But the inspiration from afar could not have been sustained and certainly not written about without the generosity of our friends at home, especially Julie Propst, who was always there throughout the writing to discuss the ideas and to help in caring for our children. As the deadline drew near and our need for larger chunks of time coincided with our children's school exams and baseball season, the kindness of our friends gave us hope to see this work through. Among these friends are Marilyn and Dick Hull, Mary Ann and Jay Fontaine, Annie Scott, Priscilla Pearson, Ruth Black, Jane and Johnny Bise, Louise and Sherman Dillon, Mernie King, Carol Tingle, Dinesh Mittal, and Alexis Polles. Some called to spend time with our children, to take the hours needed to find the special dress for Marianna, to practice batting with Van, or to tutor for math exams. Some came by to help us to take a break with guitar and good food and sang the blues. Some offered us their home or lakehouse for weekend writing retreats. Some kept us going by their own sheer enthusiasm about the work and ideas, applying them in contexts we had not yet considered.

From its inception, the persistent encouragement, wise advice, and gentle nudgings of our editors, Stephen Francoeur and Jo Ann Miller, provided the momentum needed to see the project to its completion.

Most of all, we are grateful to our children, Marianna and Van, who worked with us to create a family in which it was possible for this book to be written.

Introduction

THIS IS A BOOK about language and the body. It is written to help clinicians to learn how to use the power of language in treating patients who present somatic symptoms, whether the symptoms are considered to be medical, somatoform, psychophysiological, or factitious in origin. These problems are known by the frustration and demoralization they so often bring to clinicians who try to help afflicted patients and families. They are problems in which the occurrence or severity of bodily symptoms is governed by psychological or social influences. This book offers a practical approach for resolving symptoms that arise at the interface of mind and body—migraine headaches; exacerbations of Crohn's disease; bulimia; conversion paralysis; nonepileptic seizures; factitious symptoms; or the personal and relational suffering that accompanies chronic medical illnesses.

This work is based on an ethological understanding of language that differs from that taught to most physicians, nurses, psychologists, social workers, and family therapists in their professional training. Chapter 1 describes why failures by our medical and mental health systems to find effective solutions for mind-body problems are so significant, in terms of both patient suffering and stigmatization and enormous monetary waste in our health care system. Chapter 2 explains why so little has been accomplished, pointing to basic misunderstandings about language, communication, and the body that pervade professional training in the medical, nursing, and mental health disciplines. An alternative account of symptom generation is proposed in chapter 3 that locates the problem in social and self practices anchored in narratives of personal experience. The initial phase of a therapy—creating the kind of conversation and relationship within which important narratives can be spoken—is broken down in chapter 4 into a diverse group of clinical skills that can be practiced and learned. A detailed study of a single therapy session in chapter 5 illustrates how these principles can be put to use. Chapter 6 begins a discussion, continued through chapter 7, of what to do when the expression of personal experience is not sufficient to resolve a symptom, because the personal narratives, or self-narratives, that are available to the patient hold the body in a symptom-producing bind. One must grapple with the destructive power of these stories—at times directly challenging their authority; at other times reauthoring old narratives, creating new narratives, or locating accessible but forgotten alternative narratives that do not engender symptoms. Chapter 8 provides a more finely detailed discussion about how to ask useful questions in therapy and how to use the reflecting position to invite the creation of new meaning. Chapter 9 then provides a detailed account of an 18-session therapy, showing how the disparate parts that have been discussed are integrated into a whole therapy. Ethological pharmacology, the use of medications to create new possibilities for conversation and relationship, is presented as a more usable alternative to traditional psychopharmacology in chapter 10. Chapter 11 concludes with case presentations and a discussion of how to apply this therapeutic approach in the treatment of chronic medical illnesses.

This clinical approach evolved out of each of our personal and professional histories, since the early 1980s when we specifically focused on originating more effective clinical methods for these problems. These stories may give a glimpse of the contexts that shaped our work.

My (JLG's) father sustained head and spinal cord injuries during World War II. Through watching his quiet stoicism as he endured chronic pain, sensory loss, and muscle weakness, I learned about both the suffering of chronic medical illness and the resilience of patients and families who bear it. Later my desire to understand how minds and bodies work together took me to medical school, then to a neurology residency and neurophysiology graduate school. But I found that this understanding of neuroanatomical and neurophysiological relationships could not answer, even in principle, the questions most intriguing about my patients—how nociceptive impulses in nervous system pathways were related to the psychological reality of pain and to the spiritual reality of suffering; or how distress in a person's personal or social relationships could render his or her nervous system inoperative, as with patients presenting conversion blindness or speech loss. Well into my adult life, I returned for a psychiatry residency at Massachusetts General Hospital, where the training experiences offered were so diverse that I could study long-term psychoanalytically oriented psychotherapy, behavioral therapy, psychopharmacology, hypnosis, and family therapy with excellent supervision in each. I took each treatment approach I learned, including my neurological training, to my patients with medical and psychosomatic symptoms. However, none of the treatment approaches offered satisfactory solutions for the problems patients presented. A mix of pharmacology and family therapy seemed most promising. So Melissa and I experimented over a 10-year period with structural, strategic, and Milan approaches to family therapy, eventually settling on constructivist, language systems, solution-focused, and narrative approaches as the more fruitful sources of inspiration. The clinical approach in this book is the culmination of these repeated efforts, many of which ended in failure, to develop clinical approaches that offered patients and families more than traditional treatments could promise.

When I (MEG) was a child, I had severe asthma. As my mother, father, and older sisters took care of me, adjusting their plans when I was sick, I came to know not only the problems but also the flexibility and generosity that are possible in families with chronic illness. Later I believed that this life experience and my nursing education would prepare me well for work as a visiting community health nurse.

This was true in many ways. But the families I felt most drawn to—families whom I visited for home hospice care—found me at the limits of my skills. The individual family members, including the patient near death, would say, when alone with me, the words they longed to speak and resolve before the end. But these matters would not be spoken about when I called them all together as a family, so the patient often died with the possibility of resolution forever lost.

I pursued graduate nursing education and family therapy training in hopes of returning to hospice families to help these longed-for conversations to occur. Although I learned many theories that explained the behavior of families I had met, only through long-term psychodynamic therapy did it seem possible to relate to them with the carefulness and integrity that families of hospice patients deserved. But for hospice patients, time was of the essence. At the end of my training, I was left still not really knowing a way that would help the conversations to occur as quickly as needed. However, I did know that these wise patients, who had only days or weeks to live, and their family members, who chose to bring them home to die, each knew what needed to be spoken. I needed only to learn how to create quickly a context in which they could say to one another what they already knew. The way of working we have described in this book has been my solution to this dilemma and to many other clinical dilemmas, including that of creating integrity between my personal experience and professional thoughts and actions. I now can choose assumptions to hold about patients and families that I would have chosen to guide a therapist working with me and my family when we were experiencing the burden of asthma on our lives.

In presenting this work, we have made ample use of case descriptions and case studies in the text. The confidentiality of patients and families has been maintained by changing identifying information, such as names, ages, occupations, and locations, and by combining details from several similar cases. In some cases, such as Frances's story in chapter 3, a patient has requested that we provide an unedited story, manifesting her ongoing commitment to break the secrecy in which her former life had been lived.

We found ourselves in a quandary over the appropriate language with which to talk about those with whom we work clinically. Terms such as "patient," used predominately by physicians and hospital-based nurses, and "client," used by many psychologists, social workers, counselors, and nurses in psychotherapy practices, are heavily laden with ideological and political overtones. Although our own preferences would be to refer to those with whom we work simply as "persons," this usage could hinder, rather than help, communication. Therefore, those who are in a patient role within a medical setting are referred to as "patients" and those who are not within a clearly medical setting as "persons."

We encountered a similar quandary in how best to refer to the social unit of our therapies. Each of us works frequently with individual patients. Our preferred unit of treatment, as discussed in chapter 3, is the problem-organized system (Anderson & Goolishian, 1988), often the biological family members, although not always. For simplicity, we most often refer to "the patient and family members" as those with whom we work clinically.

Another possible point of confusion may be that of clarifying the relationship between the two of us in our work. As codirectors of a family therapy training program and collaborators in research and clinical work, we work closely together. Only in a small minority of cases, however, do we meet as cotherapists with patients or families; more often, each of us is a sole therapist. Although a cotherapist model is therapeutically effective, the clinical demands of our workplace simply do not permit it as standard practice. We each act as consultants to the other's therapy, particularly for initial sessions with families. A number of such consultations are included in the case examples presented.

In addressing mind-body problems, instead of specific diagnoses or syndromes, we are swimming against a current of disorder-specific treatments in contemporary psychiatry. This choice is intentional. Rehabilitative treatments for diverse physiological illnesses, such as diabetes, asthma, or cancer, need to be specific to the diagnosis in many areas, although even then the level of physical disability across diagnoses may be the primary determinant for treatment planning. To a more limited extent, the same may be said about Axis I psychiatric disorders, such as schizophrenia and major depression. But there is reason to be skeptical about the usefulness, at least at this point of attempting to organize language-based treatments around specific psychophysiological,* somatoform, and factitious disorders. Having worked with these problems for many years, we have found the manner in which they are distinguished in the DSM-III-R psychiatric classification to be entirely irrelevant to their practical treatment considerations. Moreover, clinicians may be wrong to expect specific treatments to emerge from future psychiatric nosologies if they accept our proposal that language influences on somatic symptoms of any sort, including medical illnesses, are mediated through emotional postures, which are general dispositions for action toward self or others. This means that the critical events in the therapeutic use of language are those involved in creating a therapeutic relationship, composing a therapeutic conversation, and facilitating the selecting and reauthoring of self-narratives that shape emotional postures (chapters 4 and 7). Although these therapeutic actions may eventually gain from more specificity for particular problems (not necessarily diagnoses or disorders), they appear to hold constant for the most part across categories of symptoms. Hence, we have taken the unconventional approach of designing a language-based therapy that can be employed across all categories of somatic symptoms, from factitious symptoms to those of medical illnesses, such as asthma or migraine headaches.

A final unconventional aspect of our work is the frequency with which we ask questions about a relationship between a person and his or her personal God, if such a relationship is significant in that person's life. Although each of us keeps a primary commitment to a spiritual approach to living, these questions are not asked for theological reasons or to probe religious beliefs. Rather, they proceed directly from the clinical approach itself.

Questions about physiology belong to the domain of relations between the self and one's body parts (neurons, neurotransmitters, hormones), whereas questions about psychology belong to the domain of relations between the self and oneself as a whole person (intentions, choices, fears, hopes) (Chiari & Nuzzo, 1988). In this sense, our questions about a person's relationship to a personal God belong to a domain of relations between the self and the embodiment, in its wholeness, of all that is beyond oneself. There can be multiple reasons why these questions are useful to ask in a therapy addressing a mind-body problem.

---

*Psychological factor affecting physical symptom, the term for psychophysiological disorders in the current DSM-III-R psychiatric nomenclature, is too cumbersome and unaesthetic and will not be employed in this text. Sociophysiological disorders would describe more accurately the symptoms with which we work but further complicate an already complex situation with unfamiliar terminology. We have opted to continue using the traditional term, psychophysiological, to refer to physiological symptoms that fluctuate with the occurrence of psychological or social events.

As Harry Goolishian commented several years ago, our asking questions about God-self relationships frequently is a way of learning and speaking the language of the patient. As such, it is an essential aspect of our effort to cast therapy within the world of meaning in which the patients and families live.

From an epistemological standpoint, the position of God in a relationship is a reflecting position as discussed in chapter 8. When a person experiences the self as entrapped within a symptom-producing dilemma, the entrapment often is maintained by an inability to view the situation from an alternative perspective that might introduce new options. A question such as: "If God were to look at this situation, what would God see?" invites a person to view a personal dilemma from a position of reflection, an observing position that frequently had gone unoccupied.

Other reasons for asking questions about relationships between the self and a personal God are more specific to the nature of mind-body problems. As discussed in chapters 3 and 4, mind-body problems are frequently organized around important intrapersonal discourse that cannot be publicly expressed with safety. That is, mind-body symptoms are closely related to secret understandings that cannot be spoken. At least for persons in Western culture with even a minimal religious life, a God-self relationship is unique in that it is the only relationship in which there are no secrets. To ask a person, "If God were to look at this situation, what would God see?" is equivalent to asking that person's most private thoughts about the situation.

The same question can also provide a unique opportunity for introducing a perspective of justice into the therapy. Mind-body problems are often consequences of the abuse of power either in personal relationships, such as spouse abuse or childhood sexual abuse, or in societal relationships, such as political oppression or racism. As chapter 3 shows, such abuses of power silence personal expression and become the ground out of which symptoms arise. The first step in therapy then is to name abuse and exploitation. For many persons, the watching eyes of a personal God provide the ultimate standard of justice and injustice. Asking, "If God were to look at this situation, what would God see?" then becomes the first step toward personal agency by claiming one's moral birthright. For all these reasons, questions about God-self relationships can offer a rich resource for therapy and are frequently asked in the case examples included in the text.

It is our hope that this book will add a new voice to an ongoing conversation. We do not believe that it displaces the pioneering work of those who worked before us with patients and families afflicted by somatic symptoms, nor would we wish it to do so. This work, we hope, will place the clinical practices of such disciplines as clinical psychiatry, behavioral medicine, structural and strategic family therapy, family nursing, and psychosomatic medicine in a fresh context that will open new possibilities. In seeking to counter the stigmatization that patients so often experience with psychophysiological, somatoform, and factitious symptoms, we hope that the book will enable more productive therapies for patients and families who have been alienated by the practices of modern medical and mental health disciplines.

CHAPTER 1

Mind-Body Problems: The Costs of Failed Solutions

MOST PATIENTS and their health care providers—family physicians, pediatricians, nurses, psychologists, social workers, and family therapists—are convinced that close relationships exist between mind and body in illness. A man with cardiac disease hears his abusive boss begin speaking and is gripped with chest pain; as soon as an asthmatic child sees her mother walk into the classroom, her desperate wheezing begins to ease; an invalid woman, chronically ill but stable for a decade, falls silent and dies within a month of the sudden loss of her husband; another woman, dying from cancer, lives against all odds until her son arrives from overseas, then dies after a last reunion. Such stories are commonly witnessed by those who care for the ill. But the nature of these mind-body relationships and how they can be used toward healing remain elusive for many clinicians.

Mind-body relationships become even more puzzling when a bodily symptom, such as abdominal pain, paralysis, or seizure, is shown to arise from an experience in the patient's life despite the absence of any documentable disease. An ambulance rushes a teenager to an emergency room, where her anxious physicians work unsuccessfully to stop her seizures by using anticonvulsant drugs. Then a neurologist examines her but concludes that her seizures cannot possibly be due to epilepsy from abnormal electrical discharges in her brain; instead, they are "pseudoseizures." Later, the patient confides to a social worker that she has been sexually molested by a family member, and the seizures stop. Manipulating physiology through pills and tablets brought no relief; yet the symptoms disappeared through talking and careful listening. Language, as this story hints, remains mysterious and is a resource not yet fully tapped in medical care.

This book is about using language to work with mind-body problems. We define mind-body problems as those human problems that can only be described through both the psychological language of feelings, intentions, and choices and the physiological language of cells, organs, and chemical messengers. Mind-body problems include symptoms seen with "illness behavior" psychiatric diagnoses, such as psychophysiological, somatoform, and factitious disorders, as well as the psychological and social problems that arise around medical illnesses. A child's diabetes that becomes more unstable when her parents fight; an elderly woman's Alzheimer's disease that leads her to accuse kin of stealing, because she cannot find where she placed her watch; the eye pain of a 10-year-old boy that is debilitating but suddenly disappears after his history test—all are mind-body problems.

There exists no general clinical theory yet that is adequate for guiding the actions of a clinician working therapeutically with mind-body problems. I (JLG) well recall my own initiation into failure: Mr. O'Malley, an obese, 40-year-old Irish man, shuffled into our Acute Psychiatry Service one summer day, sent by his internist down the hall. As a new psychiatry resident at Massachusetts General Hospital I, along with two other beginning residents, staffed a walk-in psychiatry clinic. Patients could walk into the Acute Psychiatry Service and talk with a psychiatrist without an appointment any time, 24 hours a day.

The internist had dismissed Mr. O'Malley from his office after a perfunctory physical examination and normal electrocardiogram (EKG), telling him that his chest pain was due to "stress" and that he needed to see one of the psychiatrists. Agreeing reluctantly, Mr. O'Malley had hidden his humiliation more from his internist than he did from me. Half telling the story of young deaths from heart attacks among his family members, half ventilating his contempt for the internist who had not shared in his anxiety, he talked for half an hour with hardly a breath. I listened. As I listened quietly, he settled down, evidently comforted that at least he had not been rejected. Agreeing with the internist's assessment of hypochondriasis written on the consultation sheet, I quickly formulated a plan while I listened. I would do what the internist had not done—I would conduct a thorough workup that would prove that he was not having a heart attack. Mr. O'Malley and I agreed that he would return the next time he had a bout of chest pain. I would obtain an immediate EKG while he was actually having the pain and draw blood for the heart muscle enzymes that would determine with certainty whether or not he was having a heart attack. Mr. O'Malley showered me with gratitude, barely restraining his obvious wish to hug me with affection. I was the only doctor he knew who genuinely cared about patients rather than about making money. He knew, speaking my secret hopes, that I was destined for greatness as a Harvard doctor.

As agreed, Mr. O'Malley came rushing in the next afternoon, demanding that I be interrupted from the patient I was seeing. As quickly as I could, I ordered the EKG and drew the blood studies. Mr. O'Malley insisted that he stay in the waiting room until the results could be obtained and sat for the next few hours anxiously fanning himself and twiddling his moustache.

As I had expected, both the EKG interpretation and the cardiac enzyme studies were normal. I sat down to tell him the good news. His response, though, was not as I had expected. With a demeanor more worried than ever, he told what he had read about radionuclide scans of the heart that might show a heart attack the other tests had missed. Would I order one?

Knowing that I would be too embarrassed even to raise this as a question with my internist colleague, who probably would think me a fool anyway for having done as much as I had, I decided that enough was enough. I told Mr. O'Malley that, given these normal studies, his internist had probably been correct and that we should talk about what might be happening elsewhere in his life that might so stress him that his body was showing signs of distress.

Mr. O'Malley was furious. I was a psychiatrist—what did I know? And why was I trying to treat patients' hearts anyway? Storming angrily out of my office, he half turned at the hall door to shout across a dozen waiting patients, "Go ahead and write about me in your chart, doctor, another one of your kooks!"

I had an odd mixture of feelings—fury directed at Mr. O'Malley that he had showed so little appreciation of the extra effort I had extended on his behalf, puzzlement that everything had fallen apart so quickly when it had seemed to be going so well, sorrow that he had come with a problem and I did not know what to do. He had tried to shame me in front of my other patients, yet I suspected his words were more a measure of his own shame. Troubled, I carried the story of Mr. O'Malley to my faculty supervisors. They each explained why he had acted the way he had, and I learned about patients with "borderline personality organization" and their swings back and forth between idealizing and devaluing relationships with authority figures. I was encouraged not to take any personal responsibility for what had happened but to understand his psychopathology from a position of clinical distance. No one suggested that I might have done anything differently that would have led to a different outcome. Torn between scorn and pity, I still knew that Mr. O'Malley had a problem.

As I began to discover, there is a constellation of problems that not only degrade the lives of individual patients afflicted with mind-body problems, but increasingly weigh heavily on society as a whole.

The Problem of Alienation and Stigmatization of Patients

When clinicians cannot find solutions for mind-body problems, then the patients and their families genuinely suffer from the symptoms that continue unabated. This failure exacts yet another toll when frustrated clinicians and patients reach for a target to blame. The temptation for clinician and patient to accuse each other of bad faith is nearly irresistible. Mr. O'Malley lashed out at me; it was all I could do not to respond in kind.

An inability to provide definitive relief to a patient who requests help for a bodily complaint is difficult for a clinician to bear. It brings feelings of personal failure. The feelings come close to the helplessness, anger, and despair nearly every parent has experienced when holding a crying infant who only cries louder with each effort to offer comfort. Different clinicians, of course, respond in different ways to this frustration. A local neurosurgeon, known in the community for his explosive temper, examined a prominent citizen for back pain several years ago. After he concluded from his examination that there was no physiological disease, the neurosurgeon asked his patient to bend over for one final physical examination. After the patient had bent forward, hands on his knees, the neurosurgeon swung his foot and kicked him out the door.

Patients with such somatoform problems are avoided by most clinicians. Although few act with the impulsivity and indiscretion of the neurosurgeon, probably few have never felt repulsion for patients who keep complaining, yet show no demonstrable physical disease. This aversion shows itself in stigmatizing names applied colloquially by clinicians to certain patients, such as "crock," "turkey," and "gomer" (i.e., "get out of my emergency room"). In the presence of the patient most clinicians resign themselves to working with a patient they do not like and endure the relationship stoically. But sometimes nearly every clinician loses patience.

Mr. Duquesnay was a middle-aged man with dramatic spells of losing consciousness while his arms and legs jerked. His spells were finally diagnosed as pseudoseizures, or epilepticlike behavior, occurring despite demonstrably normal brain physiology. Until his hospital admission, where specialized electroencephalographic (EEG) studies confirmed this diagnosis, his neurologists had worked intensively with him in an epilepsy clinic, trying without success to treat his spells with anticonvulsant medications. As the Duquesnay family related to me (JLG) shortly after the EEG studies:

JLG: You feel that the doctors here have not fully understood?
MRS. DUQUESNAY: [Angrily] They treat you like you don't know what you are
    talking about. They told him, "You should be able to stop them."
SON: Like mind over matter . . .
MRS. DUQUESNAY: But anybody who has watched him have a seizure . . .

MR. DUQUESNAY: Every time Dr. Day comes in, he upsets me. He says, "There
    is nothing wrong with you. It's all in your head."
MRS. DUQUESNAY: Jimmy [Mr. Duquesnay] can't stand for anybody to say he
    is faking, or he is lazy and doesn't want to work.

He, of course, could not with will power control the occurrence of his
nonepileptic seizures, and he felt as confused as did his doctors as to why
they were occurring. When I first met him as a psychiatric consultant, he was
more preoccupied with the hurt and humiliation he felt from his doctor's
response than he was with the continuing disability from his illness.

Many clinicians cannot resist scorning and avoiding patients with
somatoform and factitious problems. Some resolve to endure the relationship with stoicism and resignation. Neither response is a good one for clinician or patient.

Wasted Health Care Dollars

Public health statistics draw a disturbing picture about the incapacity of the
American health care system to address mind-body problems. This is most
visible in the economic burden of inappropriately treated patients with
somatoform and factitious disorders.

Somatoform disorder is a term used to describe patients who maintain an
unshakable conviction that they suffer from physical illness, even though
doctors can find no evidence of abnormal physiology. According to the current system of psychiatric nomenclature (American Psychiatric Association,
1987, p. 255): "The essential features of this group of disorders are physical
symptoms suggesting physical disorder (hence, Somatoform) for which
there are no demonstrable organic findings or known physiologic mechanisms, and for which there is positive evidence, or a strong presumption,
that the symptoms are linked to psychological factors or conflicts."

By definition, patients with somatoform symptoms do not experience
themselves as causing or controlling the symptoms. Mr. Duquesnay with his
nonepileptic seizures was showing symptoms of conversion disorder, one
subtype of somatoform disorder.

Patients with somatoform disorders are distinguished from those who
feel driven to commit acts to create a false appearance of illness, such as contaminating a laboratory specimen or producing falsified medical documents.
The latter patients are said to show a factitious disorder. Factitious disorders
are distinguished from somatoform disorders by the simple criterion that
factitious symptoms are conscious, willful acts, even though the underlying
motivation for the act may not be fully conscious. For example, a patient is
diagnosed with a factitious disorder when he, complaining of excruciating

groin pain, is then discovered to be covertly placing blood from a pricked finger in a urine specimen, at a time when his doctors are using the pain symptom and bloody urine as the basis for diagnosing and treating an alleged kidney stone.

A patient with a somatoform or factitious disorder often lives an existence organized almost entirely around worrying about and seeking treatment for bodily symptoms. We have encountered a number of patients with somatoform disorders who have spent $20,000 to $50,000 in a single year (bills paid mostly by health insurance). Yet, the funds expended on emergency ambulance and helicopter transports, emergency room care, hospitalizations, surgeries, and extensive medication regimens showed no evidence of resolving the symptoms—headaches, backaches, numbness, seizures—for which the patients sought medical treatment. Even when private and governmental insurance protects the patient from impoverishment from such medical bills, the expended funds intensify the stress from health care costs for society as a whole.

Systematic studies have shown that patients diagnosed with somatization disorder, a single subcategory of somatoform disorder, spend nine times as much as the average American each year on medical treatment (Smith, Monson, & Ray, 1986). Their physician visits for headaches, chest pains, vomiting, gastrointestinal symptoms, muscle and joint pains, gynecological symptoms, and fainting spells usually end in frustration for patient and clinician, because none of the symptoms respond well to traditional medical approaches. In fact, these patients not only fail to benefit from this enormous expense but sometimes are actually harmed through needless surgeries and other unnecessary tests and treatments.

Our medical systems know little about alternative ways to respond. In clinical practice, somatoform disorder and factitious disorder diagnoses are employed by clinicians more as labels to attach to patients than as useful explanations for their problems. The diagnoses provide little explanation for how the problems arise or endure—and little guidance for treatment. Although there are hundreds of published papers and a handful of books that debate how somatoform and factitious disorders should be identified, defined, and understood in clinical practice, the medical library remains nearly empty of described treatments. Carrying a general sense of therapeutic nihilism, most proposed "treatments" do not go beyond suggesting that developing a consistent, benevolent relationship with the patient is a positive measure and that one should stop patients from injuring themselves through side effects of excessive medical treatments. Among different studies, 23% to 38% of all patient visits to primary care physicians have shown only "psychological problems," with no evidence of medical illness (Ford, 1983). Although therapeutic communication is emphasized in nursing education, the problems that do prompt these lack-of-a-disease visits receive scant attention in medical education compared to attention devoted to the learning of biomedical skills—airway intubation, placing chest tubes, reading EKGs—needed in treating medical illnesses.

The consequences of this failure for public health are significant. By 1992, health care costs were absorbing 14% of American economic production and rising, threatening to add $1 trillion to the national debt by the year 2001 (U.S. Commerce Department, 1993). This stress on the economic system began eliciting calls for radical reform, even rationing of health care, from nearly all sectors of American society. Patients with end-stage kidney disease are threatened with loss of lifesaving renal dialysis because of its expense, and Medicaid funding is withdrawn from buying eyeglasses for children who need them. The problem of wasted health care dollars due to inappropriate treatment of somatoform and factitious disorders cries out for a solution. Yet, clinicians seem not to know what to offer.

Model Adoration and Model Monopoly: Small-Minded Thinking about Mind-Body Problems

A practice of "let the solution I can offer define the problem" governs how a lot of clinicians think about and deal with mind-body problems. Too few question how the implicit assumptions and the language of their preferred illness model participate in constructing what they perceive.

Physicians, including psychiatrists, tend to say about mind-body problems: "Run some medical tests. If nothing shows up, then try psychotherapy." Underlying this statement is a presumed illness model that is widely accepted among physicians: All behaviors, including mental phenomena, appear to have some physiological correlate in brain activity; therefore, all clinical problems, even somatoform and factitious problems, will eventually be explained by neurophysiology. For problems where neurophysiological knowledge is currently lacking, we will continue to try psychotherapy.

Many nonphysicians, such as psychologists and social workers, tend toward the converse approach: "Evaluate the problem as a learned behavior or in terms of its function within the family system. If nothing turns up there, or if our therapy fails to progress, we will try a pharmacological treatment."*

---

*Nurses have made more headway toward transcending a mind-body dualism. Historically, their practice has been to have sensitive conversations or to give a comforting backrub at the same time as they administer a medication. In so doing, they have been more aware of the complementarity of these therapeutic actions and have described their work less in either/or terms. However, the politics of our health care system have been such that this wisdom has not disseminated widely beyond nursing.

The situation is no different among the medical countercultures with their adherents to ascetic practices, special diets, megavitamin regimens, or physical manipulations of the body. Each claims to embody the truth about health and illness, while disparaging the worth of competing traditional and nontraditional treatments.

What is outstanding about each of these illness models is how it validates its own authority while expressing little curiosity about its limitations. Each of these perspectives, its clinical stance clearly biased by unspoken assumptions, offers a totalizing description that monopolizes the cognitive processes of the clinician. Under the influence of a model monopoly (Braten, 1987), all behavioral phenomena can be explained in terms of that particular theory: neurophysiology (e.g., "As a conversion symptom, the patient's legs are paralyzed by intense inhibition of motor systems in the brain"); psychological theory ("Positive reinforcements in the environment maintain the patient's paralysis"); family systems theory ("The patient's paralyzed legs maintain a stable hierarchy in the family by keeping her in a less powerful position than her husband"); or cultural theory from anthropology ("Her leg paralysis pantomimes a communication to her husband that cannot be spoken in words because of cultural prohibitions about roles of men and women").

As totalizing perspectives, each illness model can find some way to account for every observation, and none of the models can be disconfirmed by any observation. Therefore, whichever model is privileged by the clinician obscures any insight that the others might bring, including the models that the patient and family do bring. Likewise, a patient's favored model for explaining his or her illness obscures other possible perspectives that the clinician might bring. No feedback mechanism exists that reliably guides a clinician or patient to a correct—or most useful—perspective of what is really going on. When there is a conflict in illness model between clinician and patient, it is often resolved in the end according to which participant in the conversation holds sufficient power to impose his or her view on the other. Mr. O'Malley's anger in essence was a rebellion against a threat of subjugation that he perceived in the physician-patient relationship.

Spread across a border between the physiological and psychological domains, more than any other clinical problem, mind-body problems need contributions from multiple perspectives to be understood. Yet, tendencies toward model monopolies for understanding illness, for both patients and clinicians, erase possible contributions from any but the dominant perspective. They foster disrespect, because they render nonsensical any different perspective that might be held by another participant in the therapy. As Mr. Duquesnay and his family discovered, the world of the neurologist held no space or respect for their different perspective.

What of Other Clinical Approaches to Mind-Body Problems?

Some may object that we have overstated the failures of modern health care and psychiatry, as there exist, in fact, several therapeutic approaches within psychiatry, nursing, and psychology that attempt to accomplish exactly what we seek. They treat bodily symptoms that are not physiologically determined. They explain how mind and body interact to produce illness. A growing medical literature about treatment of mind-body problems is evidence of progress offering new hope to patients whose bodies become ill when psychologically stressed.

However, close scrutiny shows that these efforts leave much to be desired, either for helping patients with somatoform problems or for answering our personal mind-body dilemmas. In general, each available treatment approach genuinely helps some circumscribed group of patients who present bodily symptoms but not somatoform symptoms, such as those of Mr. O'Malley and Mr. Duquesnay, whose lives are largely organized around their somatic symptoms. We argue that each of these clinical approaches, although useful with specific groups of patients, shares common problems that too often disable their broader applicability, particularly with somatoform symptoms. These problems can be shown to arise out of foundational assumptions made about human beings and their language and behavior.

The Neuropsychiatric Approach

A clinician following a neuropsychiatric approach views the occurrence of somatoform symptoms as a disease, much as one would view pneumonia or cancer as a disease. During the dawn of modern medicine in the 1800s, some physicians made attempts to apply to mental disorders the same clinical-pathological methods that were proving so fruitful in understanding other medical diseases. Patients were diagnosed with hysteria when they developed symptoms of bodily illness in the absence of demonstrable physical disease (Shorter, 1992). Although specific brain lesions in specific locations could be identified in strokes, multiple sclerosis, tumors, and epilepsy, no brain lesions could be found that accounted for hysteria.

In recent years, findings from neuropsychological studies have argued that information processing in the dominant hemisphere of the brain may be awry in hysteria (Flor-Henry, 1983). Some biological psychiatrists have speculated that information transfer between the two cerebral hemispheres across the corpus callosum may be impaired in patients with bodily symptoms associated with a condition, alexithymia, in which patients supposedly do not possess language for describing inner emotional experiences (Hoppe & Bogen, 1977). However, these ideas remain theoretical and speculative and have not yet led to effective treatments organized around their principles.

Progress in neuropsychiatric understanding of psychiatric disorders has usually been evidenced by new pharmacological treatments that alter brain physiology to relieve suffering, as with depression and anxiety syndromes. Little benefit for somatoform symptoms has occurred with medications useful for symptom relief elsewhere in psychiatry, except for a subgroup of patients whose somatic symptoms are directly associated with panic attacks or severe depression. A neuropsychiatrist would find Mr. Duquesnay's nonepileptic seizures to be a fascinating form of psychopathology and would express hope that someday we will understand its underlying brain mechanisms. But this physician could offer him little concrete help.

Clinicians today generally assume that, for practical purposes, patients presenting somatoform symptoms possess an anatomically and physiologically normal brain (Ford, 1983; Shorter, 1992). The neuropsychiatric perspective, although attractive to clinicians preferring to work with a medical model for psychiatric illness, has contributed little to understanding somatoform symptoms or to relieving the suffering they bring.

The Psychoanalytic Approach

In his early work, Sigmund Freud saw libido, or life energy, as the shaping force in human behavior. If because of psychic repression libido could not be expressed through appropriate mental avenues in language or feelings, then the dammed-up libido would express itself through excessive stimulation of a body organ. Selection of the specific body organ affected would be determined by the unconscious symbolic meaning that had prompted the repression (David-Menard, 1989; Shorter, 1992). For example, a wife who repressed a wish to kill her husband for having an extramarital affair might develop paralysis in the hand that would have reached for the gun, while consciously experiencing no thoughts or feelings that would provide her with a clue as to why her hand was afflicted. Treatment then would consist of undoing the repression by providing to the disabled patient insight about the true meaning of the symptom, opening up the normal psychic channels for expression of libido.

The generation of psychoanalysts that followed Freud worked to interpret the unconscious meaning of psychic conflict bound up in such psychosomatic symptoms as hyperthyroidism, duodenal ulcers, migraine headaches, and ulcerative colitis. However, the practical results of interpreting the symbolic meaning of symptoms to these medically ill patients were for the most part poor despite long and intensive psychoanalytic treatments. By the 1950s, efforts at psychoanalytic treatment of somatic symptoms had fallen into a sharp decline (Shorter, 1992).

The Behavioral Medicine Approach

Behavioral psychologists began discovering in the early 1960s that bodily functions previously considered to operate independently from mental regulation, such as blood pressure and EEG brain waves, could in fact show learned changes. Soon thereafter, principles of learning theory were applied to a wide range of behaviors affecting health, such as weight control and smoking cessation, and behaviors influencing the course of medical illness, such as management of chronic pain and control of nausea following cancer chemotherapy. Typically, a behavioral analysis would be carried out that would identify how an undesirable behavior could be extinguished or a desirable behavior learned through behavioral conditioning.

Behavioral therapies achieved great success in regulating specific health behaviors, particularly in the controlled environments of hospitals. As a new subspecialty, behavioral medicine has developed well-defined strategies for eliminating unhealthy behavioral patterns, such as cigarette smoking, overeating, and compulsive behaviors such as self-induced vomiting with bulimia. It has designed effective methods for blocking the occurrence of such psychophysiological problems as migraine headaches by induction of a state of relaxation (Tunks & Bellissimo, 1991).

In general, however, patients who find behavioral therapies useful need to share the clinician's perspective and accept his or her guidance. This difficulty has limited the usefulness of behavioral therapies in assisting patients who do not share the clinician's perspective. Patients with somatoform symptoms typically do not share the clinician's perception of the problem and often object to the kinds of changes that the behavioral scientist views as needed.

The Biopsychosocial Model

In 1977 George Engel proposed a biopsychosocial paradigm for the organization of medical care as an alternative to the biomedical model of medical care. Engel objected to the reductionism of biomedical care that focused on a diseased organ to the exclusion of understanding the person and his or her situation in family and culture. Engel proposed that clinicians understand illness in the context of many levels of reality—cell, organ, psyche, society— as a biopsychosocial phenomenon.

Within the subspecialty of psychosomatic medicine, this perspective has provided a way to connect events in people's lives with bodily disease. A clinician can explain with logical coherence how marital distress may, through activation of the brain limbic system, alter how the hypothalamus regulates the endocrine systems and how the autonomic nervous system regulates the state of the internal organs, so that a spouse develops a bleeding duodenal ulcer, validating observations by internists decades earlier that such life-threatening illnesses as hyperthyroid "thyroid storms" and severe attacks of asthma could be triggered by fighting in the family.

Family medicine, nursing, psychiatry, and psychosomatic medicine have each found the biopsychosocial paradigm conceptually appealing. Whatever its conceptual beauty, however, its shift in perspective did not stimulate expected changes in clinical practice. In discussions, clinicians could speak easily enough about a human as a whole being with body, mind, and spirit. In clinical practices, however, translating this conviction into congruent actions became a peculiarly unsolvable puzzle.

Strong advocates of a biopsychosocial view of illness significantly influenced education in medicine, nursing, and the social sciences during the 1980s. They argued, for example, that a clinician should understand a problem, such as a heart attack, at a cellular level (how the muscle cells of the heart are injured); at an organ level (how the pumping dynamics of the heart are now altered); at the whole-person level (how the person's experience of the heart attack alters the life choices he or she makes); at the family level (how conflict in the marriage and other family relationships creates stress and a risk of another heart attack); and at the social level (how the patient reconciles the illness with productivity expectations at his or her job). A good clinician would investigate each of these levels in order to integrate them into a cohesive, multilevel description and organize a holistic treatment. Yet, the biopsychosocial approach, so obviously valid in armchair discussions among educators, had disappointingly little impact on how clinicians actually conduct themselves with patients and families. A careful examination of typical clinical encounters suggests why this is so.

Acute chest pain suggesting a heart attack is a medical emergency. A clinician does not have an infinite amount of time to gather information, nor do patients and families have an infinite amount of time and money to spend on an evaluation. Even if a clinician believes in principle that interconnected phenomena are occurring at every systemic level from a myocardial cell to a whole person to the larger society, he or she must ask: At which level will it be most fruitful to start? Or, which level, if uninvestigated, places the patient at most risk? Because there is no procedure that can provide a quick and certain answer to these questions, clinicians usually consider the problem level at which their clinical skills can be best applied according to their experience. For nearly all internists, the immediate step is to evaluate the heart as a body organ. If the EKG and other medical tests show cardiac disease, the search will likely not be taken to other system levels. Recently, advocates of a biopsychosocial model of illness have bemoaned its lack of influence in medicine and psychiatry as practiced in communities throughout the nation (Herman, 1989).

Moreover, a biopsychosocial perspective would influence the clinician to locate the pathology for somatoform symptoms in the psychological makeup of individual patients and in the dysfunctional organization of their families. Patients with somatoform symptoms, experiencing their distress in body but not in mind or relationships, feel devalued when told that their symptoms are manifestations of troubled personal lives or families and more often than not end the treatment relationship if the clinician persists with this kind of description (Griffith, Griffith, & Slovik, 1990). Although the biopsychosocial approach provides the clinician with coherent explanations for somatoform problems, many patients find the explanations to be nonsensical and humiliating.

The Shortcomings of Traditional Models: Hidden Assumptions and Constricted Perspectives

The four outlined paradigms represent the major strategies for understanding and treating mind-body problems in medical and psychological training programs. Each approach has been partially successful in providing relief of suffering for certain types of patients. Each has expanded the conceptual richness with which we can think about mind, body, and illness. However, each has fallen well short of providing a usable general theory for working therapeutically with patients who struggle with somatoform problems.

Patients' Negative Treatment Experiences

Arthur Kleinman, a noted anthropologist from Harvard University, has studied somatization of symptoms in a variety of settings in America and China. After consulting to medical hospitals for a number of years he commented on the effect that behavioral scientists have had on the care of patients presenting somatic symptoms:

> After attending these meetings for several years, I frequently came away with the disturbing impression that (at least on this service) the behavioral construction of chronic illness and disability, though frequently of therapeutic value (especially in the short run), was more demeaning and dehumanizing of patients than the biomedical model, which is so often and appropriately the recipient of these negative descriptors. As assessed by these behavioral clinicians, especially the younger ones, many patients sounded like criminals and malingerers, though few in fact actually were, and many families sounded like hotbeds of deviance propagating immoral and illegal behaviors aimed at creating havoc with the medical system. Although there was no technical reason why the operant-conditioning paradigm should lead to such a value-laden and cynical discourse on patients, that is what it amounted to. Patients were

stripped of the protection of the sick role and left in a liminal no-man's-land where neither they nor their caregivers could tell if they were morally or even legally culpable for their behavior. Once the medical category of "patient" had been undermined, these individuals, even if they had been surreptitiously labeled "crocks" by their physicians, were designated in staff-to-staff communication in a more damaging and denigrating way as "con men," "sociopaths," "deadbeats," and even worse, as faceless automatons whose headaches, back-aches, and weakness were the direct and sole result of environmental operants. Needless to say, the therapeutic discourse was no more sensitive, and you can well imagine that there was a flourishing black humor turning on the term "extinguish." (Kleinman, 1986, p. 236)

When a patient cries out in distress, over and over, that his or her body is ill or is in pain, yet no examination finds evidence of disease, does the problem lie in how the patient's brain processes information or, perhaps, with an undiscovered disease of the brain? Or is the problem located in the inner conflicts within the patient's mind? Does the problem lie with the patient's environment, which rewards these behaviors instead of other more desirable ones? Or are we obligated first to paint a more complex picture that integrates all three of these perspectives before we can look at it with understanding? These are the questions that the neuropsychiatric, psychoanalytic, behavioral, and biopsychosocial perspectives ask.

Why have these questions failed heuristically to bring forth more usable clinical tools for somatoform problems during the 100 years since Freud began his work? Clinical approaches derived from neuropsychiatric, psychoanalytic, behavioral, and biopsychosocial paradigms are, in fact, built around similar social practices, despite obvious differences in content. These similarities offer clues as to how each stumbles in a similar way when tested in clinical encounters between clinicians and patients with somatoform problems.

Clinicians' Limited Vision

If one examines the epistemological assumptions of each of the four clinical paradigms—the implicit rules that govern what constitutes valid knowledge—one can see some similarities:

1. Neuropsychiatric, psychoanalytic, behavioral, and biopsychosocial approaches each attribute little validity to the personal story about a somatoform problem as it arises from the life experiences of the patient and family members, except to the extent that these meanings fit the assumptions of their theoretical position. Stories that patients and families tell about the problem are generally discounted in favor of an expert story defined by professionals.

2. Neuropsychiatric, psychoanalytic, behavioral, and biopsychosocial

approaches all employ an unseen "bureau of standards" that has the authority to declare what is real and what is not real about the problem. This "bureau of standards," which Francisco Varela (1979) refers to as the "community of standard observers," provides an authoritative reference for valid bodies of knowledge and methodologies that distinguish between reality and fantasy and between objective and subjective truth. Therapeutic approaches judged worthy are those constructed from wisdom offered by the standard observers. However, the role of this community of standard observers is generally obscured, and their pronouncements are issued as objective facts.

Neuropsychiatrists and behaviorists look to the scientific community with its published findings from empirical studies as their community of standard observers. The psychoanalyst regards himself or herself as a person who, having completed a personal psychoanalysis and psychoanalytic education, is a qualified standard observer. The biopsychosocial clinician, trained in the traditions of medical and nursing sciences, relies both on the scientific community and the experience of the clinician to provide the needed standard observer.

However, none of these approaches includes the patient and his or her family members among the group of standard observers. They do not share the power accorded to the clinician and to the larger professional and scientific communities as experts able to define what is real and unreal. As a result, descriptions and explanations about the personal problems of patients and their family members are not a part of the professional conversation that defines what is real and what is not real about bodily symptoms.

3. Neuropsychiatry, psychoanalytic, behavioral, and biopsychosocial clinicians all use a technical professional vocabulary, such as "ego defenses," "reinforcement," "feedback loops," and "belief systems" in discussing somatoform problems. Much recent work in cognitive science has examined the powerful influence that the metaphors of language hold in focusing attention, structuring thought, and guiding the actions of users of that language. As Ernst von Glaserfeld (1988) has commented, "One cannot use a language without accepting its ontology." Yet, the influence of the clinician's professional language in shaping his or her perception and actions is hidden from their view and unaccounted for by the clinical theories that they follow. No mention is made of the influence of the trained gaze of the clinician in constructing what is seen.

For example, the neuropsychiatrist meets the patient with an objectifying gaze, in the style of an internist with a patient on an examining table, using language of hemispheric dominance, frontal and temporal lobe functions, and limbic EEG dysrhythmias. The psychoanalyst meets the patient with a studied gaze like a wise elder who has learned over the years the hidden secrets of life, listening for moments of readiness when the child may be able to hear the story disclosed, using language of wishes, fears, unconscious mind, and interpretations. The cognitive behaviorist meets the patient as a coach meets an athlete, pointing out incorrect moves and instructing correct ones, using language of behavioral reinforcement, behavioral repertoires, and cognitive distortions. The biopsychosocial clinician meets the patient as a seasoned counselor, whose diagnostic expertise comes not only from the skills from professional training but also from seeing how health problems expand outside the professional setting into work, marriage, play, and school. A biopsychosocial clinician employs this expanded version of health and illness to influence the patient and family toward healthier living, using language of wholeness, systems, system levels, belief systems, and symptom function.

It is apparent that the language belonging to each of these clinical traditions draws certain aspects about a patient into sharp focus while obscuring others. The terms of each clinical language are connected to only some possible ways of thinking about problems, to the exclusion of others. The language of each clinical tradition favors certain courses of action by clinicians toward their patients and obstructs others.

Maurice Merleau-Ponty and Martin Heidegger have spoken about the metaphors available to us in our language as lanterns that light up a small area of a dark forest (Dreyfus & Wakefield, 1988). Each metaphor can illuminate only an area of our experience, while leaving the rest in darkness. The problem is not that the languages of our clinical traditions bear this limitation (for it could not be otherwise) but our lack of awareness of what our language does not enable us to see. Each technical term clinicians use within any of the four paradigms discussed—boundaries, enmeshment, levels, reinforcement, extinction, repression, ego, drive, defense—is a well-worn metaphor that obscures from the clinician's vision the other areas it does not specifically illuminate. Because an awareness of this limitation is rarely taught in professional schools and rarely incorporated into clinical theory, clinicians from each of the four paradigms have generally lacked a curiosity about what cannot be seen with the language and cognitive style of their preferred school of practice. This lack of awareness also means that there is no avenue through which an understanding of a problem can be enriched by the unique, idiosyncratic language that patients and family members bring.

The epistemological tradition that these four clinical paradigms share forms an infrastructure on which specific clinical practices of neuropsychiatric, psychoanalytic, behavioral, and biopsychosocial clinicians are built. An analysis of this epistemological tradition suggests a direction for inquiry that can uncover why their efforts have progressed so poorly, particularly with patients presenting somatoform symptoms.

These issues are important concerns for most clinicians working with medically ill patients at home, on hospital wards, in emergency rooms, and in rehabilitation settings. Because mind-body dilemmas are delineated most starkly with somatoform and factitious problems, investigating these problems will help develop principles for guiding our broader clinical work.

CHAPTER 2

Understanding Mind-Body Problems

Mrs. CARSON, disabled from work for nearly a decade, was referred for a psychiatric consultation about her seizures. Since age 14, she would be startled regularly by electric shocklike sensations across one side of her head, then she would fall to the ground, unconscious for a few seconds. A few years later, a second set of symptoms appeared—bizarre experiences in which it was as if she were standing outside her body or that her body was numb, feeling nothing. Although she had been treated by three different neurologists over the years, the seizures never consistently stopped despite treatment trials on half a dozen different medications. She repeatedly lost jobs during her twenties because of the seizures occurring at work. At age 30, with the seizures occurring daily, she gave up trying to work. Now the family was in a crisis, because her husband had also developed a chronic illness threatening his employment. Mrs. Carson, now 45 years old, needed to go back to full-time work for the first time in years to support her family. But she was afraid to try unless the seizures could be controlled.

She saw a new neurologist at our institution, who, starting over, repeated her diagnostic studies, including observing her seizures during a stay in the hospital. He decided that her seizures must have some psychological origin; there were no abnormal electrical discharges in her brain that might account for them. She reluctantly agreed to stop taking anticonvulsant medications and to see us for a psychiatric consultation. But she and her family members were angered and humiliated by this turn of events:

[Mr. and Mrs. Carson are seated together on a sofa, with their two adult sons, Jack and Jim, seated across the room. James (JLG) interviews them about Mrs. Carson's illness and how it has affected the family. Melissa (MEG) and a family therapy treatment team are observing over closed circuit television from the next room.]

JLG: Have the four of you ever sat down as a family to talk about the seizures as a problem?

JACK: Sitting down like this? No. You know, not discussing the situation as a whole.

MR. CARSON: What are you talking about? . . . Discussing her problem in particular? Is that what you are talking about?

JLG: Yeah. That's what I was asking, but I mean . . .

MR. CARSON: Well, for us to effectively discuss that—well, that's impossible, because we're not doctors. Basically, all we can do is say: "This doctor says this, and this doctor says that." . . . End of conversation.

JIM: We don't know what's going on.

MR. CARSON: Not one of us is involved in a medical career or medical occupation of any type.

JLG: Does the whole thing seem confusing, with a lot of different pieces to it?

JACK: I don't know where it starts and where it ends.

MR. CARSON: Well, it is just like my wife told you a while ago. She agreed to be taken off the Depakote [an anticonvulsant drug]. She said, "Look. If it is not epileptic seizures, that's fine. I don't care. Just tell me what it is. You know, tell me what you can do about it—what you can do for me!" . . . That's the position, really, of the entire family. We're looking at you. And we are looking at these other professionals—medical people—to give us some answers. And, hell, you are having confusion yourselves. Can you imagine how confused we might be? . . . We get one doctor over here telling us one thing, and another doctor over there telling us another thing, and another one over here telling us something else.

MRS. CARSON: Well, I had two doctors within just twelve hours tell me totally different things. Dr. Simpson told me Tegretol [another anticonvulsant drug] won't do any good, while Dr. Major told me I had to take it for the rest of my life. I feel like Dr. Simpson doesn't want to have anything to do with me. . . . Total opposites. . . . Dr. Major says: "You need 1,000 mg of Tegretol every day." . . . Dr. Simpson walks in and says: "You don't have epilepsy. There is nothing wrong with you. You don't even need to take any medicine."

MR. CARSON: Right here in this hospital! Two different doctors . . . supposed to be the same type of doctor . . . practitioners of the same medicine . . . to tell her two different things. . . . Buddy, if that don't make you mad as hell, you're not human!

JLG: Uh-huh.

MRS. CARSON: Where does that leave me?

MR. CARSON: Where does that leave the patient? These people get paid too much money for that kind of stuff.

Despite this inauspicious beginning, the therapy was fruitful. Mr. and Mrs. Carson, without their sons, returned for 18 sessions, usually twice a month, during which Mrs. Carson and the two of them as a couple fashioned a variety of methods for eliminating nearly all of the seizures. Halfway through the treatment, she returned to full-time work as a secretary, although eventually, with the husband's improving health, the couple preferred that she take the role of full-time homemaker.

The remainder of this book describes a clinical approach for working with mind-body problems that we developed over the 12 years that elapsed since the failed treatment with Mr. O'Malley in Boston. It diverges sharply from clinical methods commonly taught to clinicians in professional schools, because it rests on different understandings of language, mind, and body from those embodied in the various medical and mental health disciplines in the 1990s.

We will return to Mrs. Carson, describing in detail the stages of her treatment, in chapter 9. Before that there are a number of questions we need to answer: How can we view language and the body in ways that are most useful for clinical practice? How can we derive a therapeutic approach from these ideas? Why might such a therapy be successful in situations where others have failed? How can this approach be integrated into one's clinical work without losing aspects of the work that one desires to keep? How can it be adapted by nonpsychiatric clinicians, such as family therapists, family physicians, psychotherapists, and nurses?

For the book to be understandable, we need to show in a stepwise fashion how our work elaborates out of a particular understanding of the relationship between language and body. To begin, we will first examine some ideas that we have chosen to guide our work and some ideas we have chosen to discard.

Ideas about Language and Communication
That Have Outlived Their Usefulness in Medicine

There are important ideas that have served the flowering of Western culture so well that they are no longer remembered as ideas but as parts of who people are. These are ideas that live so close at hand that, like body parts, they drop out of awareness. People think no more about their influence than they do about their fingers while combing their hair or about their knees while walking. It is only when they run into a problem—arthritis freezes a finger joint where it cannot grasp the comb, or torn cartilage makes every step of walking painful—that people really remember that their hands and knees have independent existences that matter in their lives. So it is with ideas.

The notion that in communication, information is transmitted from one person to another is one such assumption that is so foundational for the modern age that, like the bedrock under skyscrapers, one forgets that it is there. This objectification of information has been the foundation on which progressively more sophisticated communicational devices, from Guttenberg's printing press to television to satellite telecommunications, have been built. From this perspective, information is a "thing." Information is something created in the mind of one person to be encoded in language that is transmitted to another person, who, following decoding, receives it in his or her mind (Qvortrup, 1993).

This assumption is closely wedded to a second assumption, that language is the vehicle that carries information from one person to another. Although these assumptions about language and information are useful in designing inanimate communication systems, we challenge their usefulness for solving language and communication problems among living beings.

A computer can be programmed with a body of information. If one later retrieves the information and transfers it to a second computer, one can know with some assurance that the information has maintained a stable form before, during, and after it was programmed into the computer. In a true sense, it was "stored" in the computer, and it held a more or less fixed form as a "thing." But can one speak in even a vaguely similar way about programming the mind of another human?

Consider the case of Mr. Duquesnay. The neurologist, Dr. Day, has information, drawn from the most current scientific studies, that he wishes to impart to him about nonepileptic seizures, so that Mr. Duquesnay can correct his errors in understanding the symptoms he has experienced. Mr. Duquesnay, on the other hand, believes that he has true epileptic seizures. The neurologist will explain that scientific tests prove that his seizures are not "real" seizures but, rather, expressions of emotional disturbance, a proven fact confirmed by scientific examinations of his seizure behaviors as correlated with findings on his EEG. But this attempt to reprogram Mr. Duquesnay with valid information fails miserably, as Mr. Duquesnay not only rejects the information but also rejects the neurologist. He claims that he and his family have been traumatized by the communication. The neurologist and Mr. Duquesnay were never "in language" together. Despite using identical English words, each remained within different languages. To untangle the knotted relationship between Mr. Duquesnay and his neurologist, one had best look more deeply at the meaning of language and communication as biological and human phenomena.

By the 1970s, a convergence of two independent lines of thought—one from philosophy, another from science—together suggested a radical alternative to our traditional assumptions about language and communication, a story that begins with the life of Martin Heidegger.

How Philosophical Hermeneutics Views
Language and the Body

In 1907 Martin Heidegger, then a student in a German gymnasium, was handed by his vicar a book intended to encourage his interests in theology. Instead, the book, Bretano's *On the Manifold Meaning of Being according to Aristotle,* awakened in him a secular question that would hold his intense attention for the next 70 years: Why is it that things exist, rather than not exist? Moreover, why is it that no one seems troubled enough to ask this question? Heidegger would write 11 books about his quest of the question of Being. He would turn modern philosophy upside down, in the course recasting our understanding of language in a direction that would reveal how stories and biology connect in human beings (Steiner, 1989).

Heidegger (1962) recognized that the entire movement of Western philosophy and science since the Greek philosophers had been built on descriptions of the world made as if a human observer were in God's position, standing outside creation, not as a part of it. But every human lives in the world as a part of it, not apart from it. If one does not make this initial step of creating separateness between subject and object, between the human who describes and the world that is described, what might one then say differently about one's experience of living? Heidegger provided a detailed analysis of this immediate experience of the world—people's relationships to everyday objects used as tools and equipment, relationships to other humans, relationships to their pasts and futures, and, particularly, to our inevitable deaths.

For 2,000 years philosophers had produced system after system of tightly organized abstract concepts that rationally explained the human position in the world. Scientists had accumulated expanding bodies of facts about physics, chemistry, and physiology that could explain with greater and greater reliability how a human being operated as an organism. But Heidegger recognized that these descriptions from both philosophy and science were too timeless and too grand to capture the reality of human experience. Georg Hegel had told how history was unfolding, age by age, in a precisely logical and dialectical manner. Charles Darwin had told how nature had evolved to create the human as its pinnacle of achievement. Scientific laws had been laid down that were believed to hold as true for the atoms of our bodies as for the furthest galaxies, from the moment of creation to the most distant future. But do these grand theories help us to understand Mr. O'Malley's choice as he struggled between two alternative stories of illness—one told by the medical establishment and another told by his body in pain? Mr. O'Malley's question is a question of his Being: Who am I as a person? Am I the author of my life, or do others author my life?

Philosophy and science could each stand on their mountains and speak clearly and elegantly about humankind as an abstraction, yet say little of relevance for the deep caves of a person's specific life. Heidegger felt a strong conviction that it was in understanding plain and simple moments of everyday life, so close one might not even name them as experiences, that the secret of human existence would be found. In these moments people's deepest knowledge of themselves is that of their existence, their Being.

According to Heidegger (1949, 1962), the essence of Being is the knowledge of having two simultaneous faces, one that understands, and one that, like other objects in the world, is understood. Being discovers itself to possess knowledge of both itself and the world (including other beings) that is already given; it seems not to enter the world as a blank slate. We see this preknowledge in everyday moments: A stranger and I, having never before met, immediately agree as to which of three paintings is most beautiful; I complete a friend's unfinished sentence; at a party I catch myself before speaking words I sense would be embarrassing. When Mr. O'Malley first felt his chest pains, undoubtedly he found an immediate readiness to interpret their meaning in a particular way, although he may never have had similar pains before. How do we understand the meaning of this preknowledge in our lives? Where does it come from?

The evidence, Heidegger (1971) felt, centered on the sea of language in which people are immersed from the moment of their birth. This preknowledge is transmitted in language through both shaping by single words as they are spoken and manifold forms of idioms, teachings, prejudices, traditions, rituals, and customs that make up culture. However, this preknowledge is perhaps most characterized by the fact that it is hidden from our everyday awareness. Seldom are we aware how our questions, our manner of seeing and hearing, our curiosity have been structured out of a specific historical moment. Who could expect that either Mr. O'Malley or his internist (or ourselves) would judge his own perception of the chest pains to be anything other than an objective view, free of prejudice?

Indeed, it seemed to Heidegger that an intrinsic part of the nature of Being is that the means through which Being comes into being should be disguised. He worked for decades seeking ways to retrace the stream of Being back to its fount in language. He found the notion that people create language to be an absurd joke: People do not create language—they are created by language. In his words, "Language is the house of Being. Man dwells in this house" (Steiner, 1989, p. 127).

If this description of human existence and its relationship to language seems obtuse, it is only because it is too close and too familiar. Like the fish attempting to "see" the water in which it swims, we can't get out of it in order to see it. Or like the contoured rock of a canyon wall, we feel so little friction from the river of language that rushes by that we cannot imagine that originally it was its force that gave us our present shape. But we can identify areas of turbulence in our lives, where we can more easily feel the pressure of language in shaping our being. A specific example is the experience of speaking the liturgy for those who practice a religious life. Catholics and Anglicans recite the Mass and the Scriptures, often the same words spoken over and over, Sunday after Sunday, in unison. A Buddhist similarly may recite his or her prayers in meditation. A devout worshiper understands that something happens beyond what one would interpret to be the "literal" meaning of the familiar words spoken. As the same passages are repeatedly spoken, over and over, the language brings forth a response within the person that is unpredictable and unsteered by the intellect. This response obeys that which lies outside oneself; one becomes that which the language calls one to be. This is the heart of authentic religious experience.

It is this liturgical sense of language to which Heidegger pointed in seeking to describe human existence in its most primordial sense. One can experience the same influence of language when hearing great poetry, or, in a negative sense, one becomes aware of its power when seeking a language that remains hidden, as when one knows clearly what one wishes to say but cannot find the words with which to speak the meaning.

This view of language emphasizes, for one thing, that language cannot be understood apart from the bodily act of speaking. It describes language as the most important way in which a person can gesture, to point out to others the parts of one's experiential world, thereby creating community. It shows language to exist in the social space between persons as the amniotic fluid within which our sense of being in all its aspects—body, mind, spirit—arises. As Heidegger (1971) said,

> If we take language directly in the sense of something that is present, we encounter it as the act of speaking, the activation of the organs of speech, mouth, lips, tongue. Language manifests itself in speaking, as a phenomenon that occurs in man. The fact that language has long since been experienced, conceived, defined in these terms is attested by the names that the Western languages have given to themselves: *glossa, lingua, langue,* language. Language is the tongue. (p. 96)

> Nor is the ability to speak just one among man's many talents, of the same order as the others. The ability to speak is what marks man as man. This mark contains the design of his being. Man would not be man if it were denied him to

speak unceasingly, from everywhere and every which way, in many variations, and to speak in terms of an "it is" that most often remains unspoken. Language, in granting all this to man, is the foundation of human being. (p. 112)

We can now contrast this view of language with the twentieth-century concept of language as a "vehicle of communication." The latter perspective has been dubbed by Maturana and Varela (1987) the "tube metaphor" for communication. This viewpoint sees language as a kind of "tube" through which one person sends an idea (a communication) to another person who receives it. This model fits how computers interact when one computer sends its program codings over a cable to another computer that now stores the codings in its memory. However, in Heidegger's analysis, language is not a tool of communication, as is the interconnecting cable between the computers. Instead, it is the fundamental way in which humans are physically present with one another. Language is a way of being.

Heidegger's work pointed toward the critical importance of the ways in which language governs people's experience of their bodies and the actions of those around them when their bodies display distress. As he showed, however, this significance may be too near to them to be within their usual awareness and, hence, is not immediately accessible as an avenue down which they could seek solutions for their problems. In our day, it may be only remembered by our poets.

Even more than Heidegger, it was his student, Maurice Merleau-Ponty (1962, 1968) who saw possibilities in this line of thinking for designing a new approach for understanding problems of mind and body. He proposed that our experience of body arises in the difference between the sensations of sensing and being sensed. For example, both hands are felt to be part of the same body, a unity. However, the right hand touching the left offers the experience of body as self (the left hand) juxtaposed with self as other (the right hand touching the left one). In his words: "Once again, the flesh we are speaking of is not matter. It is the coiling over of the visible upon the seeing body, of the tangible upon the touching body, which is attested in particular when the body sees itself, touches itself seeing and touching the things, such that, simultaneously, as tangible it descends among them" (Merleau-Ponty, 1968, p. 146).

Merleau-Ponty (1964) was intrigued by the new findings of gestalt psychology. He felt that sensory gestalts marked the point of union between body and mind, a place at which subjective and objective realities touch. His perspective contrasted with a more commonly held view that we perceive the world in atomistic units of experience, like single bits of data in a computer, that are then integrated in stages to create ever more complex forms. Much of modern neurophysiology continues to be premised on this latter assumption.

For example, the neurophysiologists David Hubel and Torsten Wiesel (1979), received a Nobel prize for their work demonstrating that single neurons in the primary visual cortex of the brain respond only to specific points of light in the visual field, relaying their signals to neurons in nearby association cortex that integrate the data so that they, as neurons of association cortex, can respond to corners, edges, and lines in the visual field. These association cortex neurons, which can distinguish lines and corners, then relay their information to the inferior surface of the temporal lobe, where after further integration of information neurons are able to distinguish complex forms, such as the faces of different persons. Many, if not most, neuroscientists and biological psychiatrists assume that this stepwise organization of information processing in the nervous system, moving from perception of formless, simple sensations that are combined in stages to produce complex, patterned forms, also describes the structure of how people experience their life-world.

However, as Merleau-Ponty (1964) pointed out, gestalt studies of perception challenge whether the discovery of these neurophysiological mechanisms can provide an accurate analogy for understanding the organization of human experience. Gestalt experiments showed that we do not perceive "sense data"—isolated dots, clicks, tones, and movements that then are organized by the mind into patterns, forms, and shapes—as experimental psychologists had traditionally supposed. Rather, we often perceive complete forms or groups instead of their elements. For example, given the grouping

ab cd ef gh ij

most people pair the dots according to a–b, c–d, e–f, g–h, i–j, even though one could as easily justify b–c, d–e, f–g, h–i.

In another often quoted series of experiments, Baron Michote (1963) showed that when observers witness dots of light that are made to move sequentially in time and contiguously in space, the dots are experienced as "causing" one another to move, "dragging" one another, and "deflecting" one another. Gestalt psychology showed that people find certain primordial perceptual patterns in their experience of the world to be compelling. Perceptions are outside volitional control (body), yet they are organized in their form by a central idea (mind). If the underlying assumption of modern science is that the fundamental unit of biological information is a statement that can be coded "true" or "false" (or, "light" or "dark" in the work of Hubel and Wiesel), then the suggestion made by Merleau-Ponty is that the fundamental unit is a unit of form, a "story" so compelling it cannot be doubted by the mind or ignored by the body. Sensory gestalts are the most basic forms of such stories.

From these demonstrations of form as primary in perception, it is only a small step to argue that stories, not isolated events, are the basic units of human experience. We can call to mind, for example, important instances when perception of story is immediate, too quick to have been constructed from any discrete units of experience that could be identified and computed. Romeo catches Juliet's glance at a dance. In an instant of time he is transplanted into a narrative he cannot question and is driven to follow. (He did not pick her out of a crowd of other women by adding up points for her different features, as with a scoring system used at a beauty pageant.) A moving tree branch throws a shadow across a man's path as he steps off a subway ramp. He whirls, poised to ward off a possible mugger. (He does not conduct a detailed analysis of the size, shape, rate, and direction of the movement of the shadow in order to organize a hierarchy of probabilities for the source of the shadow.) A teacher stands before a new class of students and notes that one young man by his looks is undoubtedly a slaggard in his studies. (She does not conduct psychological testing to obtain her profile of quantified personality traits and compare it with those of studious students.) A story of passion, a story of veiled attack, a story of laziness—all these appear too quickly and in too much complexity to be constructed de novo out of primitive sensations of the moment. One can only conclude that the stories must have been already present, drawn from a canon of stories that stand ready to structure how we all experience our life-world. They shape how we perceive, how we think, how we act, granting to us a preknowledge of the world that readies us for quick action at life's critical moments. As persons, we are constituted by these stories.

There is no other part of life experience more intimate than the experience of one's body, and the security of its well-being holds a higher priority than nearly any other concern in life. There is perhaps no part of life for which a preknowledge of experience is of more crucial importance, because such preknowledge will structure one's cognitive processes to maximize speed and certainty of actions for protecting the body. If we wish to understand how another person experiences his or her body, we should begin by learning about the person's preknowledge of bodily experience. We need to know the important stories that make up a canon of first-person narratives that are available and provide this preknowledge.

One could understand Mr. O'Malley's physiological functioning through quantitative measurements of bodily phenomena, such as blood pressure, temperature, and EEG waves. From these quantitative descriptors of physiological functioning, an external observer could tell a scientific story about the behavioral phenomena observed. However, these quantitative physiological descriptors would tell nothing of the owner's experience of his body. To meet the needs of such a patient as Mr. O'Malley at the point of his life experience that will guide important decisions about his body, then one must learn how to understand the vocabulary of his experience—a vocabulary of life stories.

By definition, the task of understanding human experience is the task of hermeneutics. After Heidegger, a new generation of hermeneutical philosophers, Hans-Georg Gadamer, Richard Rorty, and Paul Ricoeur, among them, developed further this philosophical tradition that examined how body, mind, and language are related in human experience. Like Heidegger and Merleau-Ponty, they viewed an understanding of language to be inseparable from the bodily act of saying. They saw language not as a "thing," but as a way that members of a social community gesture to one another. As such, language does not exist within individual humans but in the social space between. They viewed this social matrix of language, in the form of idioms, traditions, customs, and other social practices, as creating the identity of the individual person.

In addition, their work, termed philosophical hermeneutics, showed the division between mind and body on which modern medicine is built to be a socially negotiated interpretation imposed on life as humans experience it, rather than a reflection of an objective reality that stands outside human experience (Gadamer, 1976). From this perspective, biomedical science has remained largely ignorant of its own status as one of many traditions, rather than the only valid tradition and a "mirror of reality." It has also been unaware of the extent to which its language is embodied, not in its abstract concepts and printed words, but in specific acts of clinicians talking and interacting with colleagues and patients. Thus, a biomedical clinician and a patient with a somatoform problem indeed do come from foreign-language traditions, each alien to the other in how mind and body are to be distinguished.

As has often happened during the modern age, science and philosophy marched through the mid-twentieth century with relatively little conversation between the two domains. The insights of the hermeneutical philosophers were largely outside the interests or awareness of biomedical scientists and clinicians. Their implications for medical science and psychiatry largely lay dormant. However, cognitive scientists in the 1970s arrived at a similar set of conclusions from an entirely different direction, and their work could be more easily accessed by the medical and scientific communities.

How Cognitive Science Views Language and the Body

Humberto Maturana and Francisco Varela, the neurobiologists from Chile, set out during the 1970s to understand the biology of cognition by using current neuroanatomical, neurophysiological, and neuropsychological data.

They sought to describe in mechanistic terms the causal principles that relate events that are commonly understood to represent "mental events" and "physical events" (Maturana & Varela, 1987). Their interest focused on how both "mental events" and "physical events" existed in relationship as descriptions drawn from two different language domains. What was "language" that it could constitute both the mental world and the physical world?

Staying true to their mission to provide scientific explanations in terms of structural mechanisms, they found that they could best give an accounting of language by describing it as the generation of consensual behaviors by two beings who were structurally coupled, that is, the behavior by one prompts behavior by the other in a recursive pattern that keeps the two in a stable interaction. Maturana and Varela used trophallaxis, the mechanism of communication among social insects, to help us to understand the biology of human language:

> There is a continuous flow of secretions between the members of an ant colony through sharing of stomach contents each time they meet . . . [that] results in the distribution, throughout the population, of an amount of substances (among them, hormones) responsible for the differentiation and specification of roles. Thus, the queen is a queen as long as she is fed in a certain way and certain substances that she produces are distributed among the colony members. Remove the queen from her location, and immediately the hormonal imbalance that her absence causes will result in a change in the feeding of the larvae which develop into queens. (Maturana & Varela, 1987, p. 186)

This view of language illuminated in a new way the relationship between mental ideas, language, and physical bodies as humans live together in community. Just as the social organization of the ant colony is maintained through the mutual interchange of saliva, so among humans our social organization is maintained through the mutual interchange we call language.

Both the perspective of hermeneutic philosophy and that of cognitive science point to a view of language as located in the consensual behavioral interactions between persons, not inside "the mind" of either. Rather than a vehicle that carries abstract communications back and forth between individual minds, it is a coordination of bodily states among members of a social group in a manner that preserves both the structural integrity of the social group and that of each group member.

Stories are the fundamental units of human experience and are irreducible. They cannot be broken up into more fundamental components without leaving the life-world of the person. They are the joints that couple mind and body. People do not select the stories that constitute their selfhood, nor can they easily give them up when they do not desire their consequences. These self-narratives choose us all as much as we choose them, for they are part of the sea of language within which we are all born as human beings.

Psychotherapy as a Biological Phenomenon

This view of language derived from the hermeneutic philosophers and cognitive scientists provides a starting point for designing psychotherapeutic approaches to mind-body problems that is alternative to traditional mind-body dualism. From this perspective, a metaphor is a linguistic unit of coordinated bodily states among members of a social group—a single dance step, in language, that engages the participants in interaction. A narrative, or story, is a linguistic unit of coordinated bodily states as they extend from start to end of a human experience—a completed dance, in language, engaging its participants in patterned interactions from its beginning to its end. Coordination of biological states among members of a social group occurs through the back-and-forth telling of and listening to personal stories. In a biological sense, metaphors and stories exist within the bodily interactions between persons, not as entities inside a persons's mind or as words written on paper. An example can shed some light on these concepts.

Darlene Dinkins was a young woman who requested help with severe headaches that had responded poorly to the treatment provided by her neurologist. The following is an account of one of her psychotherapy sessions.

Darlene grasped her head and neck as she sat on the office sofa. Throbbing pain had begun during our last session and had persisted all week, despite headache and pain medications. The pain was familiar, like that which for years had periodically disabled her for days at a time. She had spoken several times about feeling sad, humiliated, and angry during the first few minutes of the psychotherapy session. She did not understand why she felt this way, except that it connected somehow with the discussion we had had several days earlier about her father.

Darlene used the words "crushing" and "contorted" to describe how her head felt. She said she yearned to be "little." I asked what body position she would assume if she followed her body's lead. She took pillows from the sofa and curled up on the couch, covering herself with the pillows. I then asked what important stories from her life connected to this body position. Remaining curled and hidden, she told how as small child she would curl up like this in a closet after her father would beat her. Now, she felt deeply saddened.

Then, feeling a flash of anger, Darlene described from her teenage years an image of her father sitting in his study, in the room adjacent to the closet where she would curl up and hide. If she, in this image, were to let herself go, following the natural course of this impulse of anger, what would happen? She told how she would have gone to his closet to get his 12-gauge shotgun, then coming up behind him would have "blown his head off." Then she would have found her mother. After telling her, "You could have stopped this, but you didn't!" she would have blown her mother's head off. She remembered struggling many times with this impulse as a teenager.

I asked Darlene to look carefully about this imagined scene in her childhood home, examining her father's and mother's dead bodies splattered across the floor. What did she feel as she gazed on this scene? "Peace." I asked where she felt this peace in her body. She described "relaxation," gesturing with a hand motion from her head downward into her chest, and said that her head pain and neck cramping were both gone.

Darlene suffered under the dominion of a story that structured her body so as to bring forth suffering. For the story to endure, her body must ache. We could, of course, switch phenomenal domains and examine her body, as did her neurologist, through the lens of physiological language. With careful examination, we might then distinguish injured tissue—swollen blood vessels and inflamed muscles in her scalp, inflamed mucous membranes in her gastrointestinal tract. But rather than follow this biomedical path toward increasing scrutiny of injured tissue, we will instead refocus on the story under whose spell she lives. We will ask whether we might then find new stories that do not engender suffering.

Darlene has long since left the home of her parents, but the state of her body is governed by its place in a narrative about her father that she carries in her inner dialogue. If we are to understand her life in terms of its stories, we must first understand the characteristics of narrative language that distinguish it from other languages that also may make useful contributions to understanding Darlene's life and her pain.

Narratives are stories—"I remember when . . . " Unlike scientific language, narratives and stories have a beginning point, a middle, and a real or projected ending. The language of physiology is timeless. From a physiological perspective, we could ask about Darlene's blood chemistry, her EEG, her state of muscle tension from an electromyogram. But these quantitative descriptors are all timeless descriptors that tell us little about her temporal existence as a baby girl born into a family and a culture, who strugggled to live and grow as a child, who now is an adult looking back on those years of struggle. A human life, like a story, has a beginning, a middle, and an end.

Understanding Bodily Symptoms with a Narrative Vocabulary

By locating those critical stories that prescribe to a patient the state of his or her body, practitioners have a new way for understanding the bodily suffering the patient experiences. With this understanding, a number of questions come to mind. How can one find the stories that are most important, when, as with Darlene, they have been held so long in secrecy? Can one find ways to help such a patient as Darlene to edit her guiding narratives in a way that detoxifies their destructive power? And why should such suffering-engendering stories have come to exist in the first place? Why should anything endure at such cost?

CHAPTER 3

When Symptoms Appear

My face is a mask I order to say
nothing
About the fragile feelings hiding
in my soul.
—Mohawk Poem (Glenn, 1985)

IN ORDER TO BUILD and sustain the human relationships they most cherish, people must above all know which stories from their experience of living to speak and which to hold in silence. They must constantly guard against expressing stories that can be safely told only within private, inner dialogues.

First-person narratives ("I am . . . ," "I was . . . ," "As it happened to me . . . ") are a medium through which personal experience presses against the limitations of the social world. People enter conversations with one another based on interpretations of stories as they tell, enact, display, recite, or perform them with one another. In so doing, conversational participants are constantly reshaping, back and forth, the bodies of both self and others. But what of the times when stories of one's personal experience cannot be fitted with those of a cherished person or with narratives of a common culture that tell one how to think and to act? This sets the stage for dilemmas that cannot be expressed in verbal language but only through the body's pantomime.

The Performance of a Dilemma

Are human relationships more precious than life itself? We know of many instances where this seems so. A mother keeps her doors open to her crack-addicted son, even though he has robbed her, beaten her, and threatened her life. Marine pilots fly dangerous rescue missions to retrieve a downed pilot behind enemy lines, even though the likelihood of their deaths or capture may be greater than the likelihood of rescuing the pilot. A diabetic child in a sixth-grade class lapses into a near-lethal coma, because she feels "too different" from her classmates to follow a special diet and to take insulin shots at school.

Each person's place in the social world among family, friends, coworkers, and fellow countrymen is secured by the ability to express and to understand stories that bind him or her in communion with others. For example, two parents share with their daughter fond memories of the moments after her birth when she was first handed to them as their newborn child. They recount how she was more studious than other children, how she showed compassion to an injured frog, how she delighted her grandmother in her last years. Their daughter in turn tells of a time when her puppy was lost and her father searched for the dog until late into the night, how her mother took a part-time job so her daughter could take ballet lessons. These stories bring "family" into being.

But there are also stories that are not told. The parents do not tell about how the father had to give up plans to go to medical school, because he had to work to support the family with a new baby. The daughter does not tell how she had often sneaked out of her window at night to play with friends without her parents' knowledge. These stories could strain and threaten to sever the bonds that hold the family secure.

The same seems true on a broader social scale. Stories Americans share about George Washington crossing the Delaware River, about settlers journeying westward in covered wagons, about Davy Crockett at the Alamo, about Abraham Lincoln speaking his Gettysburg Address, all bring "America" into being. It is not surprising that efforts to introduce versions of these stories as told by nondominant cultures—Native Americans, Hispanic Americans, African Americans—into history classrooms ignite a visceral rage within many traditional Americans of European ancestry. Different versions of stories about our history as a nation dissolves some social bonds that have given shape to "America" for nearly 300 years.

Silencing one's voice in order to protect a vital relationship often makes sense, and is easily accomplished; it is much harder, yet also possible, to silence the expressions of one's body, too. Although it is difficult, people usually do learn as they grow how to disengage their bodies—their facial expressions, tone of voice, breathing, posture, and gaze of their eyes—from their private discourse, as they learn within a public discourse the ways in which they must live in order to compete in modern societies.

An incident during an interview for medical school admission has always stood out for me (JLG) as a graphic portrayal for how one may silence the body to protect a vital relationship. I was interviewing for a surgery internship at a university where the chairman of the surgery department was one of the great educators of American surgical training programs. The chairman hated cigarette smoking. While interviewing, I walked through the hospital corridors with one of the surgery residents who was attempting to sneak a quick smoke. But as we rounded a corner, we unexpectedly faced the chairman walking toward us from the other end of the hall. Without a flinch, the resident buried the burning cigarette in the palm of his hand, smiling, unhurriedly introducing me to his boss, even as the cigarette smoldered in his palm. The human capacity for creating a functional language for everyday use that is split away from the silenced body is truly remarkable.

Tom Andersen (1991) offers a beautiful description of how this shutting down of bodily expression is learned through the years of infancy into adulthood:

> A little baby moves all of his/her body when s/he laughs. The laughing movement goes out in all the body, even the toes. The toes laugh. As the child grows and starts walking, the upright position limits the possibility for the toes to take part in the laughing movement. When the child grows even bigger, s/he is taught that certain ways of laughing are more appropriate than others. When s/he becomes an adolescent, s/he may start to learn that there are things one does not laugh at, and even smiling declines.
>
> The point is that we all, including the reader, still have the potential to let the laughing movement reach and also move the toes. The possibilities only tend to be limited over time, as habits, customs, etc., are introduced. We also have the potential for even greater restriction of the laughing movement. If an unpleasant person is around, it might happen that our smiles, which previously have reached the eyes, come to stop at the lips. The unused smiles and laughs lie there, sleeping, waiting for an outburst. (p. 30)

The Process of Somatization

The splitting of language and silencing of the body seem to be the soil in which somatic symptoms grow. Arthur Kleinman (1977, 1983) in his cross-cultural studies of somatization of symptoms in America, Taiwan, and China has described somatization as a bodily idiom—a nonverbal language—that appears when verbal expressions of emotion are attenuated. In our own clinical studies we have repeatedly found patients to experience an unspeakable dilemma at the time a somatoform symptom appears or a medical symptom shows an exacerbation related to life stress.

For example, Alice Greer was a young woman admitted to our neurology service several years ago because of the sudden occurrence of paralysis in both her legs. Neurological examinations quickly established that her nervous system was intact. In talking with her during a consultation, she revealed a terrible secret: Six months earlier she had impulsively engaged in a sexual relationship with her husband's brother who was visiting in their home. Intensely guilty, she was relieved when he returned to his home in another state. But now the brother-in-law had moved to her city and wanted to renew the secret affair, threatening to divulge their secret if she refused. Unwilling to say yes, afraid to say no, and unable to talk with any person she knew about her dilemma, her legs became paralyzed, so that she could not move. Strength immediately returned to her legs as we spoke, listened, and reflected together about what she might do.

Historically, psychoanalysts became preoccupied with how such a symptom could occur without any conscious insight by Alice as to its relationship to her psychological distress. But cases we have studied, as well as others in the published literature, suggest that this is not the critical issue; the same kind of unspeakable dilemmas are a hallmark for bodily symptoms, even when the patient acts with full conscious volition to produce the symptom, as with factitious symptoms. For example, Joan Temple, a nurse, was referred for evaluation of nonepileptic seizures by her neurologist. Her situation became even more puzzling in that she also had repeated hospitalizations for kidney stones and urinary tract infections for which her urologists could find no consistently effective treatment. An interview with Joan, her husband, and her two children led nowhere: The family, the marriage, the family members as individuals were described as happy, with no troubles. In an interview with Joan alone, however, she told a secret as she wept: She had been miserable in her marriage for years, but, for many reasons, could never consider leaving it, nor could she let her husband know about her unhappiness. She had taken a lover but feared discovery of the affair. She acknowledged that she had fabricated symptoms of both seizures and kidney stones, even contaminating urine laboratory specimens with bacteria and blood, in order to appear so ill that her husband would not press his desire for intimacy. Like Alice, Joan found herself in a dilemma that, from her perspective, held no options for resolution and could not be discussed with the person (her husband) with whom a conversation must occur if there were to be any solution.

The same pattern holds even in the most extreme forms of mind-body problems. For example, Betsy Middleton was a 6-month-old baby who was repeatedly admitted to the Children's Hospital, sometimes by emergency helicopter transport, for symptoms of either respiratory distress or intractable diarrhea. In the hospital, however, the symptoms would mysteriously disappear. Suspecting a factitious etiology, the pediatric staff arranged covert surveillance of Betsy's mother, Mrs. Middleton. The next day, a nurse witnessed the mother soiling a diaper and placing it on the baby in order to create the appearance of diarrhea. Thus, the problem turned out to be that of Munchausen syndrome by proxy, a very rare factitious disorder in which a mother (as yet no cases involving a perpetrating father have been described) fabricates the appearance of medical illness in a child, sometimes placing the child at risk for injury or death. This behavior by the parent is considered criminal and is often attributed to the mother's possessing a psychopathic character structure.

However, Mrs. Middleton's situation was more complex. She was married to a much older man in a large, close-knit, and patriarchal family whose religious values emphasized a wife's subservience to her husband. Recently, Mrs. Middleton had been raped by her husband's brother. Although her husband and the entire extended family were angered by the brother's action, they agreed he should not be banished from the family home, because "he was family." They also insisted that no mention be made of what happened outside the family, because it would sully the family name in the community and their church. The brother-in-law continued to visit Mrs. Middleton's home, making what she perceived as sexual advances toward her. She found the Children's Hospital to be a safe haven away from her family and the brother-in-law, but passage to this haven was only granted by the sickness of her baby. Again, Mrs. Middleton was presented with a dilemma for which she could see no solution, and about which she could not talk with persons who possibly could help her.

In these kinds of dilemmas, a person feels trapped, not only because there is no obvious avenue for solution, but also because the kind of conversation essential for its resolution cannot take place. As such, these dilemmas resemble double-bind communications, although of a special sort. The double bind was described by Gregory Bateson's research team in 1956 as a communication in which: (1) There is an instruction on one level of communication; (2) there is a simultaneous instruction on another level of communication that conflicts with the first; (3) the recipient of the communication is forbidden to comment on the conflict; and (4) the recipient of the communication is forbidden to leave the field of interaction (Bateson, Jackson, Haley, & Weakland, 1956; Sluzki & Ransom, 1976). The unspeakable dilemmas of mind-body problems are double-bind situations in which the patient attempts to resolve the situation by silencing his or her bodily expression of distress. While the final mechanism remains a mystery, a somatic symptom seems then to occur as the body escapes efforts to suppress its expression. But understanding this terminal event in symptom generation is less a concern for the design of a therapy than understanding and intervening in the social context that triggers the symptom—the unspeakable dilemma.

Of course, there are a multitude of different perspectives from which one could ask other sorts of questions about how such symptoms arise. From a neurophysiological perspective, one could investigate how dissociation (the phenomenon of splitting consciousness into more than one part or of selectively shutting down certain capacities for the body to sense or to move) occurs neurologically, or whether conversion symptoms in humans are homologues of the freeze reaction, or immobility reflex, seen in other animals when trapped. From a psychoanalytic perspective, one could ask, as did Freud, whether intrapsychic conflicts and unconscious motivations produce somatic symptoms. From a behavioral perspective, one could inquire how somatic symptoms arise and are maintained through positive reinforcement in the patient's environment. From a religious or moral perspective, one could question how sin or ethical violations can play a role in generating such symptoms. It can be argued that each of these perspectives, as well as still others, is valid and asks valid questions within its domain of discourse. A better neurophysiological understanding of somatization, for example, might provide an explanation for why some persons never show somatic symptoms, even under conditions of extreme distress, whereas other persons show them immediately.

Our purpose here, however, is to find a better way to use language for resolving mind-body problems. For our ends, some perspectives are more useful than others. The one we have found to be the most generative is the study of a mind-body problem within its context of language-organized social interactions: We focus on the unspeakable dilemma—the double-binding situation—in order to understand it and to seek ways for the patient or family to escape it.

Unspeakable Dilemmas Are Anchored in Critical Life-Narratives

In each of the three discussed examples, there was from the patient's perspective unavoidable entrapment (no options for escaping the dilemma) and isolation (no possibility for the kind of conversation through which a solution might possibly be fashioned). So why couldn't any of these three persons locate options for a solution that had gone unseen or, else, find a way to begin the needed dialogue about the dilemma? Why are patients and families unable to find more productive perspectives from which to view their double-binding situations?

One can return to Heidegger's insight that language, not people, is in the driver's seat. What one can see, what one can think, what one can act upon are governed by the language in which one lives. The specific implication of this insight is made clearer by examining how language—as a storied experience—is related to everyday emotion, cognition, and action.

In a biological sense, an emotion is a dynamic disposition of the body for action (Maturana, 1988), that is, an emotion of fear is a readying of the body to flee; an emotion of anger is a readying of the body to attack; an emotion of sadness is a readying of the body to search for what has been lost. This understanding of emotion differs somewhat from the common vernacular in which emotion is considered to be synonymous with feeling. From a biological perspective, a feeling is an immediate way of evaluating and monitoring one's emotional state, but it is not itself a primary component of the emotion. This view of emotion follows a line of anthropological, sociological, and physiological research extending from Charles Darwin to Humberto Maturana. It leads to the definition of a new term, emotional posture, as a way of explaining how life-narratives contribute to the endurance of unspeakable dilemmas (Griffith & Griffith, 1992a).

First, an emotional posture is the overall configuration or patterning of body components that, during a specific emotion, participate in readying the body for a specific path of action. An emotional posture refers to both components traditionally considered mental (such as shifts in focus of attention or level of vigilance) and components traditionally considered physical (such as changes in heart rate and muscle tension). To inquire about an emotional posture, detailed questions are asked that identify the physical positioning of the body and the specific bodily sensations that are experienced, followed by a question such as: "If you were to think of your body as getting ready for a particular kind of action or a particular kind of expression, what would that be?" In this inquiry, one could well omit asking for the name of a feeling that would describe the emotion. For example, the emotional posture of Joan Temple, in the previous example, could best be described as a bodily readiness to hide.

This biological view of emotion holds several specific benefits for the design of therapy for mind-body problems. First, it provides a way for simultaneously describing a mind-body problem in both linguistic, psychological terms (the patient's life story) and nonlinguistic, physiological terms (brain systems for information processing). In chapter 10 we discuss how this dual description provides a framework for coupling "talking" and medication treatment, so that the two different approaches can complement and potentiate each other.

Second, patients who appear for treatment often are emotionally malfunctioning in that their feelings no longer provide an effective monitoring of emotional state. If during childhood acclimatization has occurred to harsh emotional environments, for example, a patient may no longer experience angry feelings in situations where his or her body shows physiological signs indicative of anger and where others in the culture typically would describe angry feelings. Through understanding the body's emotional posture, however, one can nevertheless work directly and accurately with its emotional state, even while bypassing discussion of feelings.

Third, this understanding views emotion not as an individual event occurring in isolation within one person's body but as an interpersonal event within a social field. This perspective opens many new possibilities for therapeutic actions within the relational world of the patient.

Fourth, our focus of attention on emotion as readiness for action, rather than the feelings experienced, keeps us oriented toward finding specific ways in which a patient and family can act, rather than feel, together in order to escape a symptom-producing dilemma. Too often, traditional therapies have been preoccupied with analyzing the problem, rather than planning a way to escape it.

Emotional Postures and the Generation of Somatic Symptoms

The silencing of bodily expression in mind-body problems entails holding one's body suspended within a particular emotional posture, readied for an action that never arrives. If we had seen Mrs. Middleton in the midst of her predicament, we would have seen her terror when faced with menacing approaches of the brother-in-law who had raped her juxtaposed with the neglectful absence of protection by her family. Her racing heart, tensed muscles, wide pupils, recoiling body posture, and scrutiny of his movements, together described a coordinated preparation of her body for flight. But she did not flee, and the outward signs of terror were camouflaged as she went about her daily housework and meal preparation, as if the brother-in-law were not in the house. What blocked her flight?

We turn to the stories she had available to guide her life in order to understand. Particular stories from her lived experience—her self-narratives—collectively provided for Mrs. Middleton a sense of selfhood ("I must be the kind of person who is . . . "). For example, she vividly recounted stories of growing up as a little girl during her mother's three marriages, witnessing her mother being beaten by men and living in homes where there was little protection offered to women and children. There were stories of her own numerous illnesses as a sickly child, during which the kindness of nurses and hospitals offered an occasional haven from her chaotic home. These self-narratives prescribed that she should camouflage her terror from her family members and acquaintances, expecting that no one would respond protectively to it. The plots of her self-narratives pointed toward a single avenue for escape, seeking patienthood under the care of doctors, nurses, and a hospital. Fabricating the appearance of illness in her baby was simply a means to this end.

In addition, there were influences from other kinds of stories whose sources were outside her personal experience. There were religious stories about "Wives, be subject to your husbands as though to the Lord" (Eph 5:22–23). There were stories from a patriarchal rural culture about men's rights to pursue pleasure from women. There was a notable absence of cultural stories about women receiving community support in defying a man. All these were cultural narratives into which she was born, that formed part of a social matrix through which she understood the meaning of her life as a woman, a wife, a mother. These stories offered no direction for her to move in her terror. The stories from both her intrapersonal psychological world and her interpersonal social world provided no options for action and simultaneously forbade meaningful dialogue with those persons—her husband, other family members, friends, community law enforcement authorities—with whom a conversation conceivably could have created a path out of her dilemma.

Self-Narratives and Beliefs Are Different

One may wonder why we have referred repeatedly to the influence of stories or narratives, rather than to that of beliefs, in fostering mind-body problems. After all, cognitive-behavioral therapists, as well as family therapists (Wright & Leahey, 1987), have developed methods for changing patient and family belief systems deemed pathogenic for a patient's symptoms. Although clinicians often use the terms interchangeably, there are in fact significant differences between a patient's (or family's) stories and a patient's (or family's) beliefs, and quite different clinician-patient relationships evolve depending on which is used to conceptualize the problem in the therapy.

Fundamentally, a story is the immediate experience itself as organized temporally within language. A belief, on the other hand, is an abstraction, a summary description of those aspects of a story, or group of stories, that are important for guiding future action. A story approximates "what happened" as immediately experienced; a belief is an interpretation and a reduction of that storied experience. Mrs. Middleton's stories about staying in bed with stomachaches and headaches until she was taken to visit the kind family doctor or about witnessing her mother's beatings by the stepfathers, each were situated in a certain place, at a certain age of her life, and with specific characters in the story. From these bundles of stories she carried into adulthood, she drew certain beliefs to apply generally to all life situations: to expect men to abuse women; that one's family offers no protection against abuse; that doctors, nurses, and hospitals will care for and protect you. In a therapy with Mrs. Middleton, does one work with her beliefs or with her stories?

In our work with mind-body problems, addressing beliefs instead of stories can be problematic for two main reasons. First, the therapy attempts to work collaboratively with patients and family members in creating new linguistic distinctions about mind and body that enable a revision of current stories of mind and body. This way of working aims for change in the quality of experience itself. Although a change in beliefs naturally ensues, the clinician attempts to freely follow, rather than to guide, the patient in interpreting their new beliefs from the new stories.

Second, a clinician can only serve as a consultant to a patient in reconstructing the patient's story, as only the patient can access this immediate experience. Beliefs, on the other hand, are similar to opinions in that there obviously exist multiple interpretive possibilities. Whereas a story is compelling in its immediate presentation, beliefs are much less so. Beliefs can be challenged. Consequently, clinicians working with beliefs tend to work from a more authoritative, challenging stance with a patient or family. In our approach we search for a consultative, reflective position, from which questioning emerges out of genuine curiosity, a "not-knowing position," as Anderson and Goolishian (1992) have described it. It is easiest to maintain this position as clinician when talking about immediate, storied experience, rather than the beliefs drawn from it. These differences are summarized in table 3.1.

TABLE 3.1

Differences between Self-Narratives and Beliefs

Narratives or Stories	**Beliefs**
1. Stories involve fundamental distinctions about mind and body.	1. Beliefs involve how experience organized by these distinctions is interpreted.
2. Stories are specifically situated in temporal experience.	2. Beliefs are timeless abstractions from storied experience.
3. A personal story is compelling, hence unassailable. Its acceptance does not demand rational justification.	3. The existence of a personal belief, as an interpretation, implies the possibility of alternative beliefs. Beliefs require rational justification, even when based on religious or philosophical faith or dogma.
4. Only a patient can speak with authority about his or her story, because only the patient holds access to the immediate experience.	4. The possibility of rational alternative beliefs immediately raises questions about true or false beliefs and who has the authority to make this distinction.
5. Therapies based on stories of experience evolve toward collaborative and consultative relationships between clinician and patient (or family).	5. Therapies based on systems of beliefs evolve toward the clinician's holding an instructive, authoritative, or argumentative position in the relationship between clinician and patient (or family).

Why Some Life Situations Are Both
Unspeakable and a Dilemma

The treatment approach presented in subsequent chapters is organized by an understanding that (1) persons are bound by unspeakable dilemmas in part because of the specific narratives they have available to guide their actions; and (2) other new (or revised) narratives can help them to escape these dilemmas.

There are a variety of explanations—some intrapersonal and psychological, others interpersonal and social—why certain narratives prevent a patient from escaping a dilemma generating bodily symptoms. Some of these explanations describe difficulties some persons have in composing usable stories—the critical areas of personal experience may be inchoate, with no language available for talking about the experience with others. Other explanations describe intrinsically destructive ways in which personal narratives and social practices in the culture can interlock. The latter include (1) the ways that certain kinds of personal stories forbid one's experience to be shared with another person; (2) the ways that some stories carry such destructive consequences for the self or other that they cannot be safely spoken; and (3) the ways that certain social practices of the culture prescribe a dilemma, while forbidding conversation about it.

When One's Experience Is Inchoate

A person can lack the emotional vocabulary and the needed linguistic distinctions necessary for articulating one's life experiences in narrative form: "I don't know what I feel," and "I don't feel anything," were frequent comments made by Ms. Martin, a young woman referred for treatment of intractable headaches. A full history revealed that her headache problem was only one from a batch of somatic symptoms—abdominal pains, blurry vision, backaches, dizzy spells—about which she chronically complained. She found herself perplexed and unable to complete a home record for documenting how severe her headaches were during different days and situations, because she literally did not know how to grade them on a spectrum of severity.

She had grown up in a home where relationships had been primarily functional ones and there had been little talk about or expression of emotions. Much of the therapy focused on slowly creating a personal language with which she could learn to notice the details of her bodily experience and express them in words.

We can say that, in truth, Ms. Martin experienced life but did not know what she experienced. She could only know that for which she had language available for knowing. Success in therapy for her lay in building a language with which she could speak—with herself and with others—about her mind and body. As Edward Bruner (1986b) has said, we cannot understand our experience when we have no language with which to understand it; and, when we do not understand what we are experiencing, we are helpless when we attempt to communicate the experience to others.

When Life-Stories Forbid the Sharing of Personal Experience

Narratives can be destructive if they hold as an assumption that sharing one's lived experience with another is either impossible or dangerous. Such an assumption entrenches efforts to suppress bodily expression that are so closely connected to the appearance of somatic symptoms.

For example, Mrs. Jackson's admission to our psychiatric inpatient unit was prompted by a suicide attempt, slashing her arms and taking a drug overdose, that occurred during a bout of severe headaches. She had had daily headaches since a head injury years ago in a motor vehicle accident, and they had improved little with the usual medical treatments. Careful study of the pattern of her head pain suggested that some worsenings of her pain related to how she experienced communications with close friends and with her husband. It was, however, extraordinarily difficult to talk about these matters, because her stated conviction was that, "Things are better if you keep them to yourself."

As Mrs. Jackson's life-story unfolded, she told how she had been regularly abused as a child and had married at a young age in order to get out of her home. She grew up experiencing herself as an unwanted child whose presence seemed to have caused trouble in family relationships whenever she had been noticed by the others. As a child, she often said to herself, "Things are better if you keep them to yourself" and "You had better keep your mouth shut."

Mrs. Jackson's dominant self-narratives were composed in childhood as stories about a little girl whose visible presence only seemed to upset family members. These self-narratives actively hindered the kind of talking needed to make any headway in improving her head pain.

When Life-Stories Are Too Terrible in Their Consequences

Some narratives are intrinsically destructive, because they propose to solve a problem by negating, or eliminating, either oneself or another person. Such stories are often so threatening that they are held in secret.

After months of individual psychotherapy, Frances, in treatment for bulimia, revealed a plan for stopping the sexual abuse in her family that she had long held in secrecy: "About all of the sexual abuse. I cannot tell my mama. She couldn't handle it. She couldn't hear it and it would make no difference anyway," said Frances. "I must suffer this alone. Only God can really know my pain, and he understands that I may have to die. He will take me home."

Frances appeared to be well on her way to dying at 80 pounds, wasting away from bulimia, with severe chest pain and blackouts. "But something, someone has to stop the cycle of abuse," she said. She knew her nieces and other young women in the family were now being abused, too, and often, as her own had been, the abuse was ignored. "In my dying, in my final silence, they will hear. It is the only way to stop it. There's no other way they will ever realize how destructive the abuse is."

Frances was bound by a powerful narrative that called for her death as a solution for the sexual abuse in her family. In therapy, the answer to her dilemma might seem obvious: Frances should confront her mother with the secret that had obstructed her recovery from bulimia. But this belief belied the deadly accuracy with which Frances understood the power of the secret in her family.

While she was in the hospital I (MEG) asked to meet with anyone in her family that she would allow me to. Not her mother—that was understood—but her two sisters came, one of whom had also suffered childhood sexual abuse. Frances and I told them that the secret was so strong that it might kill her; that she felt that under no circumstances could she tell their mother, even though it might save her life, because her mother was too fragile to hear it. "What are your thoughts as you hear this? Do you understand that Frances feels her life is entrapped in the dilemma?" I asked her sisters, knowing they would be bound to say that she must tell. Perhaps they would even feel that everyone in the family would somehow benefit from breaking the secret. But I was stunned by their response, "We understand—and she's right—Mama must not be told. We love Frances, but she has to do what she has to do. We have already bought her a cemetery plot. We hope she doesn't do it, but we don't blame her. We do understand." It was very painful to have her sisters make way for her death, but Frances began her preparations, writing a letter that her mother was to read after Frances died.

In time, she did not die but found her own way to escape the power of the secret. The change did not occur within the conversations of her therapy sessions but within Frances's conversations with her personal God. "God can do lots more with me than you can, Melissa," she said. In an about face, she took the risk of writing her mother a new letter, forgiving her, but asking her mother to acknowledge all the years of sexual abuse that she was certain the mother already knew about. Her mother acknowledged that abuse occurred and expressed regret that it happened. Frances felt this was not fully the response she desired, but it was enough.

Once the secret was broken, Frances's self-narratives underwent revision, saying: "The truth, not death, can set me free." Soon after, she began to conquer the bulimia that had dominated her life and her body for 18 years. The story of a fragile mother who required the sacrifice of her daughters for her own sustenance was transformed into the story of a relationship between a mother and a daughter that outstood the winds of tragedy.

When Social Practices Prescribe Dilemmas But Forbid Discussion

The lens selected in presenting most of the preceding examples has been person centered. The unit of study was each person as an individual considered together with his or her life-narratives. This lens does not draw into focus the social contexts within which each patient lived and out of which his or her life-narratives were born.

Each of the examples could have been considered differently. A social-constructinist lens would have shown, instead, how social practices—customs, idioms, habits, fads, rituals, institutions—shaped these lives and their narratives, so that symptoms appeared. In this manner, social practices can both create human dilemmas and regulate whether there can be public discussion about the dilemmas. It is useful, then, to examine different kinds of social practices and how they provide a context for the appearance of mind-body symptoms.

If one thinks about where and how different kinds of binding narratives arise, one can devise a sort of typology of social practices from which narratives that bind the body are born. Of course, a patient stuck in a dilemma quite often can be viewed as stuck in the middle of multiple binding narratives of different kinds, all working together to hinder moving toward a solution. We also acknowledge that divisions among these types of social practices are to an extent artificial, in that each division is a linguisitic construction that tends to spill over into the others.

For example, we told the stories of Alice Greer, Joan Temple, and Mrs. Middleton differently, by organizing them around the psychiatric and psychopathological diagnoses of the individual patients—conversion disorder (Alice Greer), factitious disorder (Joan Temple), and Munchausen syndrome by proxy (Mrs. Middleton). When using such psychopathological nomenclatures, clinicians are preoccupied mainly with how best to classify patients according to the pattern of symptoms expressed. But this attitude leads to a therapeutic dead end and has thus far proven of little practical use for clinicians treating patients and families. Organizing stories according to the social practices instrumental in creating dilemmas provides a quite different way for understanding them that leads directly to solution scenarios. In order to capture the complexity of ways in which social practices can create binds upon the body, we will examine a variety of different social practices.

A Typology of Binding Social Practices

Political Directives That Bind the Body

Explicit political directives can place a person in such a dilemma that suppressing expression—both voice and body—seems the only safe course to follow. Such directives create a dilemma through the threat of violence and the fact that talking about the dilemma is illegal.

Consider the following description by Nora Gallagher (1991) of life in Czechoslovakia following the 1968 Soviet invasion, based on her interview with Petre Bos, a Prague family therapist:

> Routes of escape from family life that we take for granted were rarely available to people in Czechoslovakia. Travel was either forbidden or complicated (mandatory sessions with the police attended one's return and travelers suffered from "border nightmares") . . . . The interior of the family was stressed and there was a hidden panic that the family could or would fail or break. . . . I think there was a lot of psychosomatizing. I suspect social and psychological problems are hidden in a lot of ill people.
>
> Outside the family, a protective disguise was necessary: some pretended to be good party members; others withheld loyalty but were careful not to confront. The adaptation process to a totalitarian regime resulted in public mistrust, paranoia, pretending, false compliance, anxiety, and creating a false social self. . . . We belonged to the conspiracy of pretending. It was a culture, a need to survive, to keep the family intact and to survive socially. (p. 52)

Similarly, Carlos Sluzki has provided accounts of family life in Argentina during the days of military dictatorship when 10,000 to 15,000 of its citizens became "the disappeared," victims of torture and murder when informants reported to authorities that their words or actions were suspect. During this time of terror, armed military and parapolice squadrons would suddenly appear during the night at the home of a suspect. After breaking down the doors, the armed men would blindfold the suspect, then drive him or her away in unmarked cars, sometimes taking their family members as well. Those taken would seldom be seen or heard from again. During the abductions, any witnesses or family members would be told: "If you mention anything about this to anybody, they [the one abducted] will be killed immediately. If you keep total silence, you may see them again." In this passage, Sluzki (1990, p. 137) writes about a family whom he interviewed in Buenos Aires, in which the parents of a troubled child were among "the disappeared":

> I turn to grandmother, "Ma'am, I would like to have your perspective. How has the health of this family been, as you see it?" This question triggers a collective roar of laughter. Grandmother states, "During these last two years it has

been a major disaster, just an interminable series of things! First, my former husband got cancer. Then my gall bladder acted up. Then my husband got sicker and died. Then came the accident of the kid [referring to the sailor], with his arm in a cast for a year, graft surgery, and the lot. Then, after his accident, I had a gastric hemorrhage due to an old ulcer reactivated by medication I was taking for my arthritis, and I was in bad shape. And also the little one [referring to uncle/daddy] has a swollen ganglion that has to be biopsied in order to find out what's going on. Summarizing, health is a big disaster. And my daughter, with all her worries about the kids, everything she eats upsets her stomach." Uncle adds, "We all have ulcers in this family. I also have an ulcer in the duodenum." I comment, "So, you are a family of worriers." The girl adds jovially, "And we kids have indigestion and colitis." Grandmother concludes, "Since two years ago we haven't had any respite."

As Sluzki then commented, "The intense psychosomatic displays of this family seem to replace the expression of, and dialogues about, an emotional pain that is as unspeakable as the losses from which it stems."

In nontotalitarian, Western societies, we find remarkably similar examples of somatic symptoms that have been fostered within micropolitical systems of abusive families, where a child sexually abused at home hides the abuse at school and church, even defending her father as if he were a wonderful parent; or where a wife is physically beaten at home by her husband but hides the abuse even from friends or coworkers, believing that she cannot or should not escape and will only suffer more if she were to disclose.

Sexual abuse, specifically, is so commonly identified among children who present to emergency rooms with nonepileptic seizures that its possibility must be considered in every case, as the following example illustrates.

Thirteen-year-old Jana had been referred to a neurologist colleague after she had been taken from school to her local emergency room on three occasions for seizures. At school she suddenly fell from her desk and began jerking her arms and legs and writhing on the floor, later denying any memory for each episode. The consulting neurologist quickly identified the spells as nonepileptic seizures, and demonstrated he could trigger them by giving Jana an injection of saline (a salt-water shot as a placebo) together with words suggesting that the shot would cause a seizure. He reassured the patient and her mother that the spells were not neurological seizures and did not require anticonvulsant medications.

In meeting with Jana alone, however, the story widened. With specific questioning about possible abuse, she told how during the summer, while out of school, she stayed at home with her stepfather on days that her mother worked. When they were alone, the stepfather had sexually fondled her and warned her not to tell anyone. She had not spoken out of fear that she would not be believed, that she would be punished by him, or that the revelation would threaten her mother's new marriage. She was terrified that he would touch her again but spoke to no one. Instead, her body began jerking violently, out of control.

Like Julia in George Orwell's *1984*, victims of political oppression may learn how successfully to show a public face and to speak public words that satisfy those who hold authoritarian power—"If you kept the small rules you could break the big ones"—all the while running a black market of private thoughts and felt emotions that bear no relation to the public presentation of self (Orwell, 1949, p. 107). No doubt, this strategy is essential to survival in dread situations. However, its cost is the stressing of mind and body in a way that creates optimal conditions for somatic symptoms.

These accounts linking political oppression and somatization are instructive, because they strike down an unfortunate legacy of psychoanalytic thought according to which intrapsychic, unconscious processes are central to the generation of somatoform symptoms and treatment of these symptoms requires new conscious awareness of these intrapsychic conflicts. In the treatment of Anna O. that gave birth to psychoanalysis, for example, Josef Breuer (Breuer & Freud, 1957) encouraged her stream of free associations and retrieved from her unconscious a conflictual memory of her struggle during a sexualized dream against a snake attacking her sick father. His understanding was that her symptoms improved as she gained insight into her unconscious processes and traumas buried there, whereas Sigmund Freud viewed her symptoms as symbolizing her repressed sexual attraction to her father. It is likely that neither Breuer's nor Freud's interpretations pointed to critical events. As Breuer discovered, "The things she told me were intimately bound up with what was most sacred to her" (p. 43). More likely, Anna's act of speaking openly her sacred, private language shattered the bind that required its secrecy. Whether or not she had "insight" into her conflicts prior to meeting Breuer is uncertain and may have been of little consequence. After all, she had already described her free associations to him as her "private theater" (p. 41). Now her private theater became public.

This emphasis on insight and conscious awareness has been unfortunate, because its influence has pushed to center stage in clinical settings the kinds of questions that surround and plague patients presenting somatoform and factitious symptoms: Is the patient doing this on purpose, or is it unconscious? Can one help the patient to gain insight into the psychological nature of his or her symptom? What might the repressed conflict be that could produce such a symptom? Such questions both pathologize unnecessarily the patient and also shift the focus of treatment away from a far more productive avenue—first, determining which real-life dilemmas and the narratives they have birthed have bound the patient in such a way that expression is shut down; and, second, helping the patient to find concrete ways to get out of the binds.

Political decrees prescribe dilemmas, yet explicitly forbid the subjects to express how they experience their dilemmas. The Czech families described by Bos, the Argentine families described by Sluzki, and Mrs. Middleton who fabricated the appearance of illness within her baby, each possessed insight about their dilemma; the problem did not represent a lack of insight but a lack of free expression. The problem is the dilemma and the stories attached to it, not the patient or the patient's mentation.

Cultural Practices That Bind the Body

There are cultural practices that prescribe dilemmas, while forbidding the kind of conversation needed to resolve them. Less overt than intimidation through violence, they nevertheless lock persons into similar kinds of binds.

Binding cultural practices arise from societywide narratives about gender, race, age, economic status, or ethnicity that explain what it means to be so labeled. Participation in important social networks can depend on whether a person can constrain his or her bodily expression according to the dictates of the group requirements for membership.

Although illustrative examples are easy to find within any of these categories, the role of gendered social practices in producing somatic symptoms among women is a particularly timely topic.

Mrs. Smith, a 32-year-old woman, was admitted to the hospital agitated, threatening suicide unless something were done to stop her headaches. She described a crescendo of frustration due to medical expenses that were burdening her family, because concurrent treatment by a neurologist and a psychiatrist had failed to stop her head pain. Little further history could be obtained, other than from medical records supplied by her physicians, because she was so distraught.

As she neared the end of a 4-day regimen of heavy sedation, her head pain diminished enough that she could tell the story of her pain. She felt tormented by her headaches, because they always seemed to come on when she was trying hardest to prevent them—when sitting at her daughter's piano recital, going out with her husband on their anniversary, preparing a family dinner at Thanksgiving. The more she would think, "I'm afraid I can't make it!", the more upset she became, judging herself to be a failure as a wife and mother because of her headaches. Finally, she voiced a secret about which she was deeply ashamed—her husband, sober and a hard worker during the week, was a binge drinker on weekends. When drunk, he was irritable and aggressive, at times grabbing her hair and twisting her neck, or banging her head into the wall, once breaking out teeth. She blamed herself "for being such a bitch" and for her shortcomings as a spouse because of her headaches.

Among Mrs. Smith's extended family and church acquaintances, it was understood that "boys will be boys" and cannot be expected to meet the same standards of consideration of others as can women. There was also an unspoken assumption among other family members that problems in the marriage were bound to be caused by her too-frequent illnesses. She did not wish to pursue family therapy, because she felt that she would be stigmatized in her community for shaming her family through such a disclosure to an outsider.

Mrs. Smith's story seems anachronistic in places where feminism has had enough influence that protesting wife beating is the expected norm. But even among the culturally sophisticated, there are some kinds of gendered constraints that can create binds as unspeakable as those endured by Mrs. Smith—magazine ads and television commercials that specify how women's bodies should be shaped; traditional standards for training in professional education that grant no time for parenting children; implied threats of dismissal from work if there are complaints about sexual harassment.

The telling of one's personal story is no less a political event in democratic societies than in totalitarian societies, no less for Mrs. Smith in a small American town than for Petre Bos in communist Czeckoslavakia. The anthropologist Edward Bruner (1986b) concurs in his writings about political struggles that are expressed through different national myths and rituals among a people. As he notes, "The ability to tell one's story has a political component; indeed, one measure of the dominance of a narrative is the space allocated to it in the discourse" (p. 19). Whether in societies or in families, alternative stories competing with a dominant story of the culture are not granted "air time" within accepted forums for discussion. They must seek expression through underground and unorthodox channels of communication. Allocation of space in public discourse is thus one of the most important aspects of power distribution in society. For Mrs. Smith, an alternative view of marriage that would challenge her husband's conduct could not be placed on the table for family or community discussions; its expression could occur only through the underground theater of her body and its illnesses.

Authentic expression of personal experience is always fluid, idiosyncratic, and unpredictable. It does not know the bounds imposed by cultural practices. It inevitably takes a stand against some type of cultural practice, except in those rare locations where an ideological commitment to open dialogue guarantees space for many different kinds of stories and values each of their expressions. A therapy session should carry such a commitment.

Religious Practices That Bind the Body

There are religious practices that prescribe dilemmas, yet forbid the kind of conversation that would be needed to resolve the dilemma. Wencke Seltzer (1985a, 1985b), studying children with conversion symptoms in the National Hospital of Norway, noted that to an unusual extent families whose children presented conversion symptoms were highly moral, often active in fundamentalist religious sects. This focus on normative moral categories of right versus wrong and good versus bad seemed to abort the expression by family members of their individual life experiences. As Seltzer noted, "Generally, feelings were converted and sorted under the family's moral code. These were reduced to normative categories of good/bad, right/wrong, etc. . . . States of discomfort, anger, pain, and sadness were seldom expressed verbally" (p. 275).

Religious practices closely resemble other cultural and family influences in their shaping of bodily expression—with one important difference: Among Western religions, authentic religious experiences involve intrapersonal dialogues with a personal God that are privately held. These are perhaps the most privately held of all conversations that a patient may bring into a therapy room. Hence, they are often kept outside the awareness of a clinician unless deliberate inquiry is made. Yet, they can hold great power for freeing or constraining the body.

For example, Betty Varner brought her 11-year-old son to therapy. "He won't mind, and he won't go to school. Lord knows, he's got good reason to have problems, but this won't do. I've prayed and prayed for Jack—I can't discipline him, and I can't see that he's any better."

She asked for some moments to talk alone. Jack asked if he could please leave. "I can't stand to see my mama talk about what she's about to tell." I (MEG) accommodated this mutual request. Jack left the room, and Betty explained why she believed Jack was having problems: He, his brother, and his cousins had all been repeatedly raped by his father several years ago. When Betty learned of this, she confronted her husband, despite his threats to her own life. She had him arrested by the sheriff, testified against him in court, and saw him sentenced to the state penitentiary. However, this act gave her no sense of absolution. She felt she should have known earlier about the abuse, so that it never would have happened or gone on so long.

As she told about the abuse, her breathing speeded, quickening to such short, shallow breaths that she was gasping and trembling. She became pale and started to rub her left arm, which was causing her intense pain. The paper bag I offered her was not of much assistance; I understood now why Jack had wanted to leave her. "This just happens. I don't want to talk about his dad anymore. Now you know. I'll be OK."

As her breathing returned to normal, I asked about what had been happening with her body. "It hurts. My heart hurts the most. Sometimes I think I am having a heart attack. I wish I would, then I could die, but I never do."

"Do you talk about it with anyone else?" I asked.

"My church friend—she is my best friend. We go together to church three times a week. Sometimes we pray together."

"And do you talk with God about this?"

"Oh, no! I never talk about this. I pray a lot but always for other people. See, I can't ask for God's help, because I haven't forgiven my husband. I know I am supposed to forgive him, but I just keep hating him. I know I'd kill him if I could, and I can't go to God unless I've forgiven him. No, I've heard my preacher say . . . and the Bible says . . . you can't ask God for help until you have forgiven . . . so I can't. Maybe that's why I hurt. Maybe God gives me this hurt, so I can hurt like my babies hurt when they got raped. I want to hurt. I wish I could hurt as bad as they did, but I know I don't."

It would seem that for Betty to find relief from her hurting, she must live within a story where her God can listen to her anger, yet does not inflict pain on her heart. If one could carefully create a therapeutic relationship that shows both reverence and interest in her intrapersonal dialogues with her God and in her interpersonal dialogues with her pastor—perhaps including the pastor in her therapy—then openings to new stories that would comfort rather than afflict her body might become possible.

Family Myths That Bind the Body

Some family myths also prescribe dilemmas while forbidding the kind of conversation needed to resolve the dilemma. Among 15 families whose children showed conversion symptoms, Wenke Seltzer (1985a) noted a high prevalence of shameful family stories from past generations with themes of poverty, alcoholism, or social stigma. Awareness of this "heritage of damaged goods" appeared to have pressured the parents' striving for normality, propriety, and uniformity within the family while avoiding talking about the stigmatized past. Children in the families encountered expectations that they attain a level of academic or athletic achievement that would restore lost honor to the families but for reasons left unspoken. In this family context, the children became disabled from symptoms of paralysis, pains, hearing loss, and mutism.

Families are small cultures with their local myths about "who we are as a family." When the strain between expressing "who I know myself to be as a person" and "who we are as a family" becomes too great, it invites the same splitting between public (family) expression and private expression that we have already discussed.

Mrs. Merton, for example, appeared in our office at her internist's insistence after he concluded that her episodes of abdominal pain and diarrhea were largely stress related. Mrs. Merton, a 25-year-old mother of a 2-year-old daughter, was working full-time while also taking graduate art courses at night. She told a story of a long-standing struggle between following the path of her family and that of her own heart. Art had been a deep source of joy in her life since childhood. Quite talented, she had won art scholarships and awards during college.

Her excitement about art disturbed her parents, however. They told her stories about her father's uncle, a black sheep in the family who had been an artist with an explosive temper, deep mood swings, and periodic psychiatric hospitalizations. To the relief of her parents, she switched college majors to accounting during her last year, and now had a successful accounting practice. Unknown to them, however, she was now finding her work as an accountant to be tedious and empty and still entertained private fantasies about leaving it someday to return to her art. Her symptoms later improved as she began to voice openly her discontent and to create a place in her life for art.

In order for her to escape the bind upon her body, it was necessary to name the family myth about her uncle that still held sway over her family life, to identify the places in her life where it held power, and to stand in opposition to its influence.

The Silencing of Expression Is as Important as the Dilemma Itself

A survey of these examples shows each to qualify as a double-bind situation, with some additional features added. Double-bind social situations associated with somatic symptoms are those for which the patient's attempt to escape the dilemma is through silencing the spontaneous expression of bodily distress.

Detailed interviews of patients suffering from somatoform symptoms have shown that the bodily experience of such a dilemma is that of mobilizing the body for action (e.g., an aggressive emotional posture), while expressing a contradictory emotional posture (e.g., a warm welcoming, with smiles and attentive listening, belying privately held seething). In essence, the body receives two conflicting directives for organizing its physiological readiness to act.

Thus, it is not the intensity of a powerful emotion, such as anger, fear, or shame, that typically triggers a somatic symptom; it is the effort to silence the expression of anger, fear, or shame that usually triggers the symptom. From an ethological perspective, this is a "command to camouflage" the body's emotion, homologous perhaps to the "freeze reaction" or immobility reflex that other animals show when threatened in a trapped position. One cannot *not* perform socially—when performance is forbidden, one offers a somatized expression by the body as the *performance of a dilemma*.

For example, Mr. Ames was a 50-year-old man diagnosed with "hysterical weakness" of his arms by his neurologist. He had been frightened, believing he was having a stroke, when he became unable to move his arms and hands following an argument with some neighborhood children. Ill with emphysema and recovering from depression, he had felt tired after mowing his lawn. While he was resting, two fourth-graders playing nearby turned up their jam box loudly. Mr. Ames asked them to turn it off. They complied but appeared in Mr. Ames's opinion to mock him. He was enraged but checked his impulse to grab them by their throats. Shortly thereafter, he became barely able to move his hands and arms.

When interviewed in the hospital, Mr. Ames detailed his bodily experience of the incident:

MR. AMES: Before I knew it, I came close to tearing them apart. I could have choked both of them. Of course, I talked to them later and apologized. It hurt me to know that I was capable of that.

JLG: But you said you were trembling and shaking. What did you notice was going on with your body after they left?

MR. AMES: I felt a flooding, a flushing, a burning come all over my body. I guess my blood pressure was up.

JLG: Was it how angry you got or that you were getting angry and trying to stop getting angry both at the same time?

MR. AMES: It was not in my nature to do that. I could feel my nature taking over . . . "Stop! You shouldn't be doing this. This is not you." I could feel that.

JLG: With these kids, when you feel the rage to hurt them and at the same time yell at yourself, "This is not you!" . . . what is it like to be caught between those two sets of feelings?

MR. AMES: It seems like a war going on inside my mind.

The Postmodern Age and Binding Dilemmas

The dilemmas that bind the body appear to afflict more people today than in past eras, with the possible exception of the Victorian age. For the Victorian period, the prevalence of somatoform symptoms was blamed on the repression of sexuality. However, at least among heterosexuals, this could hardly be the case today. It seems strange that so many people would feel so trapped in an age best known for its cultural permissiveness and freedom of expression. The dilemmas of our age are different. Typically, they are characterized by experiencing oneself as "having no voice," a theme that is now dominant among many psychiatric problems reaching epidemic proportions, such as eating disorders, alcohol and substance abuse, and chronic sequelae of sexual, emotional, or physical abuse in childhood. There must be some reasons why somatic symptoms would occur in so close relationship to the experience of "having no voice."

There is seldom space for voices of whole persons in the discourses of contemporary society. Today it is common for many persons never to feel known as a whole person anywhere. We all live in a world of flux, of rapidly shifting functional relationships. For example, I (JLG) vividly recall how certain my identity seemed while growing up in the 1950s. I remember walking through a forest on a gravel road about 10 miles from my home in Prentiss, Mississippi, when I was 12 or 13 years old. A man in a pickup truck stopped and asked me who I was. "I'm Lamont Griffith's boy." He nodded and drove away. I realized then that I could go anywhere within Jefferson Davis County and would be known as "Lamont Griffith's boy." My identity was spread securely over 1,000 square miles of unchanging earth. Few of us today, myself included, can now claim that certain sense of personal identity.

Moreover, emotions of intimacy in past generations were reserved only for committed relationships that endured endlessly despite the changing circumstances of the participants' lives. But now emotions of intimacy are without lasting commitment—in psychotherapy sessions, at Club Meds, at health clubs, in transient coworker relationships in offices. This freedom, however, has also brought a consequence: People often find themselves known only in their parts, one part of their person for each relationship that finds that part useful for its needs. They may change their relationships as quickly as they move from one apartment and one city to another, following a job and occupation. In this flux and complexity of relationships and the rushed lives people live, they often know one another only in a partial way while pretending it is the whole. Increasingly they live with a sense of being known only in one dimension.

"Having a voice" seems to be a code phrase for "expressing who I know myself to be." As discussed, many mind-body symptoms arise out of dilemmas of expression—if I show myself as I know myself, then I fear I will no longer fit within this relationship I must preserve. I risk losing either the relationship or my sense of selfhood. I may be spewed out; I may look in the mirror but see no one. Mind-body symptoms are the performance of this dilemma.

Other have made similar observations. The Harvard psychiatrist Arthur Barsky (1988) has written about the decline of social institutions that in past generations aided the ill and suffering—neighborhoods, extended families, religious communities. As persons become estranged from one another, a sense of vulnerability grows, often focused on one's bodily vulnerability to illness. Without these rich social networks and the opportunities for dialogue that these relationships bring, it is difficult to protect oneself from the divisiveness of modern life that renders difficult the discovery of the wholeness of life. James Fernandez, professor of anthropology at Princeton University, proposes that the central problem for our age is how to maintain a sense of wholeness in the face of the atomization and economic individuation of modern life. Flooded with more information and more communications than we can possibly assimilate in a thoughtful manner, we often relate only at our lowest common denominators—a McDonald's menu of shared life experiences. Consequently, we are better understood, Fernandez notes, "as 'dividuals,' rather than 'individuals,' negotiating multiple and often incompatible memberships in separate self-contained associations" (Fernandez, 1986, p. 160).

In a fascinating book, *The Managed Heart*, the sociologist Arlie Hochschild (1983) uses the training experiences of airline flight attendants to illustrate how postindustrial capitalism has come to rely on the buying and selling of emotional labor, or feeling management, as "the management of feeling to create a publicly observable facial and bodily display" (p. 7). Flight attendants, who are trained to maintain a warm, friendly, pleasant demeanor no matter how hostile or obnoxious a plane passenger may become, find such selling of one's expression to lead easily into a habitual objectification of self, as a robotlike, detached, alienated experience of oneself. Hochschild voices her concern that exploitation of emotional labor by corporations and national institutions in our day is leading to a widespread and intolerable estrangement of workers from their feelings and from their bodies. When one is paid to manage one's expression of feeling and body so as to fit the expectations of whichever stranger walks in the door, the split between public and private discourse is complete.

In a sense, people live now in a place of permanent frontier. Lives of high mobility, where traditions, market demands, and authorities mingle and compete for influence, rely on ad hoc negotiations to determine what should stand, for the moment, as acceptable social behavior. Whether one can risk revealing wholly oneself in these rapidly shifting relationships seems to stand as a question that must be asked over and over. A season for dilemmas that cannot be spoken but only performed is upon us.

CHAPTER 4

Language and Emotional Postures

IF WE ARE ON TARGET in viewing a somatized symptom as the public performance of an unspeakable dilemma, then we should expect the freeing of expression to relieve a person's symptom. Furthermore, if specific life narratives are the glue that holds such a dilemma in place, then reconstructing these life-narratives ought to loosen the bind. Treatment of a somatized symptom logically should start by creating a kind of conversation and relationship that invites a person's and family members' personal expression through the telling of important stories of lived experience. This step alone may bring dramatic relief when the silencing of personal expression has indeed been the primary obstacle to the resolution of a symptom.

But how does a clinician create such an invitation? By what skills does one create a conversation in which what has been unspoken can be heard? Answers appear as one looks more closely at complex interactions among domains of emotion, knowledge, and expression in the social formation of mind-body problems and then works backward from them toward a solution.

Creating a Biological Context for the Telling of Personal Stories

Mr. and Mrs. Mason sat politely with their children. Mrs. Mason had been admitted to the hospital because of a sudden paralysis of the right side of her body, now much improved. Her neurologist had diagnosed the paralysis as a conversion symptom. Although she had improved spontaneously after admission, he felt that there were unaddressed problems in the family and insisted that she see a psychiatrist. In meeting each family member, I had the following conversation with her daughter, Nona, age 14.

JLG: How have you talked about our meeting today? What conversations have you had?

NONA: [Speaking for the family] The doctor says that Mother was under a lot of stress, and that made her sick.

JLG: Did that sound to you like a good reason for us to meet or not?

NONA: In some ways it did, and in some ways it didn't.

JLG: What were some ways it did not seem like a good idea?

NONA: I think there are some things that aren't anybody's business but those in the family.

JLG: I agree. If I ask any questions here today that seem to be intrusive, or about things that are just family business, then say you want to "pass" on that question. I'll go on to another question. I think we can do everything we need to do here today just talking about things people are comfortable talking about.

This vignette shows how emotional postures can either open or close possibilities for therapeutic dialogue. All mammals, including humans, show two broad groups of emotional postures. Emotional postures of tranquility are the different configurations of a bodily readiness to care for oneself or another. For mammals without language, these include grooming, grazing, playing, among others (figure 4.1). Monkeys play at the zoo, hardly mindful of strangers watching; deer graze in a pasture, heads lowered while gazing at the ground.

Humans show the same emotional postures of tranquility, as well as others that language enables, such as reflecting, composing, listening, musing, affirming, understanding, trusting, loving. Old friends chat quietly, rocking on a porch, while time slips away; a child curls up with a book on a sofa, oblivious to the sound of her mother's voice calling. In emotional postures of tranquility, attentiveness to controlling one's physical environment is minimal. In particular, vigilance to threat is low. Attention is focused inwardly on oneself or on one's inward resonance with, or understanding of, another person. In a relationship, one enjoys the touching, with paws or hands or words, by the other.

Emotional postures of mobilization, however, are different configurations of a bodily readiness either to defend or to prey on. For mammals without language, these include stalking, guarding, attacking, glaring, hiding. A cat, barely moving, quietly stalks a bird; a rattlesnake, beating a rhythm, coils to strike a leg that comes too close. Humans also show these emotional pos-

Figure 4.1

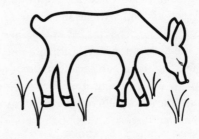

TRANQUILITY

Without Language:
**Grooming, Grazing, Nurturing,
Digesting, Resting, Gazing, Playing**

With Language:
**Reflecting, Listening, Wondering,
Creating, Musing, Fantasizing, Day-
Dreaming**

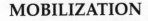

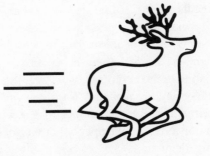

MOBILIZATION

Without Language:
**Exploring, Investigating, Showing
Alarm, Mobilizing, Readying to Attack
or Defend, Stalking, Fleeing**

With Language:
**Justifying, Scorning, Shaming,
Controlling, Distancing, Protesting,
Defending**

tures, as well as others that language enables, such as scorning, shaming, blaming, criticizing, justifying, walling off, ignoring. In emotional postures of mobilization, the perceptual, information-processing, and motor systems of an organism are primed for controlling its environment. Vigilance for potential threat is high. Attention is focused outwardly in an effort to predict and to control the behavior by one's prey or adversary. In a relationship, touching is either entrapping or threatening.

In nature and in human society, there is a liminal zone in which an organism scans the environment in search of signals for alarm, while remaining for the most part in a state of tranquility. A grazing deer may look up, prick its ears, and sniff every few moments, before returning to the grass to eat. Birds roosting may sit quietly until a human approaches within a precise distance, upon which they burst into flight. Ethologists have referred to this "flight distance" as the animal's umwelt, the proximity within which an intruder will trigger alarm. Among humans there have been many studies about territorial space, as in experiments in which the investigator repeatedly tests how close a stranger on a subway or in a public library will permit the investigator to approach before showing alarm. There often is a precise and predictable distance past which the approach of a stranger will trigger defensive behaviors (bodily signs of readiness to fight) or fearful behaviors (bodily signs of readiness to flee) (Goffman, 1971).

For humans with language, an umwelt is shaped by social practices—the customs, habits, idioms, rituals of a culture—that give a sense of safe and unsafe territories of discourse while communing with other humans. There are thus some personal stories that can be shared with most persons, others only with selected persons, and some with no other person without risking the triggering of alarm. This watchfulness can be seen as the Mason family members present themselves. In the room everyone was smiling and cordial, with the parents encouraging their children, "Don't hold back. Say whatever you are feeling." Yet, there was a tenseness of the faces and tightness in the laughter that bespoke a vigilance for potential threat. Although only Nona spoke openly her wariness, it was no doubt shared by each family member.

Psychologically, a zone of alarm governs the degree of intimacy in conversation and in relationships. Outside the zone of alarm, one can socialize with tranquility; when its terrain is transgressed, however, an alarm is triggered, followed by fear or anger or emotional withdrawal. Permitted topics of conversation; how quickly (if ever) certain personal facts are revealed to a stranger; which expressions of which emotions may be witnessed by which persons; whether one can look directly into the eyes of the other; all are testimony to a zone of alarm that is largely bounded by expressions of language.

Being Aware of the Constraining Impact of Emotional Postures of Mobilization

Emotional postures of mobilization can effectively imprison a person within a symptom-producing dilemma, because they compound two separate processes, each of which diminishes the person's and family members' capability for solving problems. First, an emotional posture of mobilization is a reflexive withdrawal by the whole organism from a painful situation. This withdrawal, for humans, includes the isolation of private discourse about the problem from conversations with other persons, including those from whom aid conceivably could be obtained. Second, emotional postures of mobilization are, physiologically, a reconfiguring of perceptual, information-processing, and behavioral brain processes that maximize the speed and efficiency of response, while minimizing the creativity and complexity of response. Emotional postures of mobilization are an aid when one struggles alone; they are a hindrance when depending upon cooperation within an intimate relationship, such as that between patient and therapist.

How Emotional Postures of Mobilization Isolate Private Discourse

Life narratives that constrain bodily expression arise in relation to binding social practices. In the usual discourses of daily life, verbalizing such narratives would breach the silencing that has been prescribed by the binding practices. This abrogation entails the risk of stepping into a zone of alarm that would trigger emotions of shame, rage, fear, sorrow, or other expression of pain. These emotional postures of mobilization, as a self-protective movement by the body, camouflage and hide the life story.

Expressing these hidden narratives thus occurs only when an atmosphere of safety can be created that does not ordinarily exist in spontaneous everyday discourses. Creating this safety zone is the responsibility of the clinician. The difficulty of this task is often not understood by novice clinicians, who wonder: "If this secret is causing so much trouble, why not speak it and get it out of the way?" An emotional posture of tranquility signifies that enough of a sense of safety exists for this to feel possible.

How Creative Problem Solving Is Hindered by Emotional Postures of Mobilization

Emotional postures govern access to knowledge, because they bias perception, patterns of cognition, and possible actions. As part of a coordinated readying of the body for action, neurophysiological systems anticipate what information will be needed for guiding the expected actions. Perceptual systems—seeing, hearing, touching, smelling, tasting—are then sensitized to detect this specific information. Related patterns of thinking and acting are also prioritized. For example, moving shadows, sudden sounds, and footsteps immediately catch one's attention, but while walking through a dangerous neighborhood at night, the beautiful old architecture and the romantic glow of the rising moon pass unseen. The body is attuned only to possible signals that warrant flight.

Taken together, these cognitive readjustments create a high likelihood that certain kinds of information in the environment will be noted and other kinds of information ignored. We term this resetting of information systems an epistemological stance (Griffith & Griffith, 1990, 1992). An epistemological stance is the relationship between an emotional posture and the kind of knowledge that it renders accessible to a person. Because of the readiness it brings for noticing and responding selectively to events, each emotional posture prescribes a specific epistemological stance. In the Mason family interview, Nona's epistemological stance was one that attended selectively to aspects of my communications that could be threatening. She would have been "unable to hear" reassurance from me.

This relationship between emotional posture and knowledge access is critical for understanding human relationships. For example, partners in most dyadic relationships, such as marital or clinician-patient relationships, tend to drift into emotional postures that complement and stabilize one another. This implies, however, that the couple partners will tend to notice certain kinds of information but tend to ignore other kinds, depending on the epistemological stances of the relationships. When an epistemological stance tends to preclude information that is essential for solving a relationship problem, the relationship can become stuck in an impasse.

In clinical settings, a mind-body problem is usually associated with a particular dominant emotional posture. Often, this emotional posture structures an epistemological stance that obscures the knowledge needed to escape the dilemma. This is particularly the case when the dominant emotional posture is one of mobilization. Because emotional postures of mobilization selectively focus attention on a feared external threat, often, this very vigilance hinders escape from a dilemma, because it sacrifices opportunities for noticing unexpected events, reflecting thoughtfully, thinking creatively, and opening oneself up to new, more adaptive ways for solving the problem.

Using Language to Foster Emotional Postures of Tranquility

Quite simply, a clinician's skill in enabling patients and family members to tell their personal stories consists of skills for helping another person to enter emotional postures of tranquility, despite unavoidable ambiguities in the therapy situation that could plausibly signal a threat. The narratives on which the success of therapy for a mind-body problem hinges are those that bind the patient within an unspeakable dilemma. These narratives are hidden by the splitting of public and private discourse under threat of punishment, shame, or sorrow. They can be spoken only when safety and protection are guaranteed. The telling of important personal stories and emotional postures of mobilization do not coexist.

Much as the skilled host of a dinner party can, by careful selection of guests, wisdom in the arrangement of seating, and artful turning of the conversation, enable conversations to occur that might never have taken place spontaneously, so can a skilled clinician enable the kind of conversation through which patients and family members can devise escapes from binds that bring on symptoms. However, doing so requires special skills. We group these skills into three categories:

1.) Structuring a clinical setting for a therapeutic conversation that invites the telling of personal stories.
2.) Using language to construct a conversational domain for talking about personal stories.
3.) Engaging oneself in the conversation to open access to knowledge.

Structuring a Setting for Therapeutic Conversation

Over the years we have developed guidelines for structuring a meeting among clinician, patient, and family members that engenders such emotional postures as curiosity, respect, and openness. Insofar as these guidelines address questions of power and control, they also constitute a political stance for therapy. They can be grouped into four general categories that are not mutually exclusive: Protecting the integrity of personhood of the participants; establishing egalitarian relationships; taking into account the impact of the clinical setting; and taking into account the relational impact of the clinician's expert knowledge.

PROTECTING THE INTEGRITY OF PERSONHOOD OF THE PARTICIPANTS

Clinicians should take active steps to protect the integrity of personhood of therapy participants. As with the Masons, clinicians usually should begin a session by asking the patient and family members only to answer those questions that they feel comfortable with. The work to be done can be conducted with only what can be spoken without duress or in response to interrogations. In addition, clinicians should inquire whether this kind of meeting to discuss personal or family business with a professional is a brand-new experience. If so, they should be sensitive to the possibility that it may be enough at this session simply to get to know one another (Andersen, 1991). When working with an observer team of therapists, we usually negotiate the structure of the session according to the preferences of the least comfortable family member. For example, he or she may wish that our colleagues be present with the therapist and family in the therapy room, rather than having the team observe the session over closed-circuit television as is our more common practice. Or he or she may wish that the team make recommendations following a discussion outside the therapy room or that they discuss their observations as a reflecting team in the presence of the therapist and family members (Andersen, 1987b, 1991).

When meeting with a family, we most often pace the interview according to the most hesitant family member. We often think about families in the way Maturana and Varela (1987) describe herds of antelope. A herd of antelope on the grasslands of Africa can appear to be surprisingly at ease, heads down grazing, oblivious to any danger. But if one looks closely, there stands at the edge of the herd an antelope with head up, demarcating the umwelt, watching. A signal from this antelope sentinel and the entire herd vanishes in a flash. When meeting with a family, it is always most tempting for a clinician to talk most with the member who seems most open and comfortable with talking in order to get the greatest volume of information the fastest. But our clinical work is about creating conversation through which a new world, not yet known, can be discovered, not about gathering information about an old world organized around the problem. We prefer to be guided in our work by the bodily stance of the most hesitant family member.

We find this attentive courtesy for safety and comfort of the patient and each family member to be essential for reflection and creativity to occur. We find our most useful principle to be Tom Andersen's recommendation always to move "from the usual to the less usual, not to the unusual" (Katz & Doyle, 1986, p. 7). In his words:

> In order to stay in a conversation with a person, one must respect the person's basic need to conserve his integrity. In order to be able to do that, one has to learn to be sensitive to his signs, which often are very subtle indications that our contributions to the conversation have been too unusual. One thing that helps to see these signs is going slow when talking with people, i.e., going so slow that they have time to let us know their responses, and we have time to notice them. . . .
>
> Sometimes a person engages himself in a situation that at this point in time represents something that the person is not ready to take part in. The mind has not yet been able to understand what this might be. But the body has. The body gives its signs that there is something in the situation the person should be pro-

tected from at this point in time. The body has grasped the idea about this, which the mind has not yet. (Andersen, 1991, p. 26)

ESTABLISHING EGALITARIAN RELATIONSHIPS

Clinicians should strive to establish egalitarian relationships within the therapeutic conversation, while openly acknowledging the power differences between clinician, patient, and family members inherent in the structure of therapy. This therapeutic approach strives to restore a unity of language in which mind and body, public and private discourse can be rejoined. Hierarchies of power in human relationships tend to silence the nondominant participants. It is therefore important for our therapeutic efforts to create therapeutic relationships that are as egalitarian as possible, with each participant in the process participating actively in decision making.

Although submission and deference by patients and families to their clinicians are obstacles best cleared away, this ideal is never achieved in practice. Habitual ways of meeting as clinician and patient in a professional office or hospital, negotiations about goals, the payment of fees, who talks and who listens all are social practices prescribed by our culture. Embedded in these practices are assignments of skills and power to the clinician that are not accorded to patients and families. In addition, clinicians cannot escape the implications of gender, race, socioeconomic class and what these distinctions can mean in the therapeutic relationship.

Some clinicians, with good intentions, minimize or deny the significance of such clinician-patient differences, but this seems only to leave the patient mystified. Patients and family members who experience differences, such as race or gender, as powerful realities may yet feel it necessary to submit to the clinician's authority by pretending a collegiality that does not in fact exist. Such collusion then becomes one more form of public and private discourse splitting within a relationship.

It is important to seek mutual respect and acknowledgment in clinician-patient relationships; it is also important to express honestly the unavoidable power inequalities that do exist. There are a variety of measures for protecting an egalitarian relationship while acknowledging these inequalities.

The expertise of the clinician can be defined as that shown by a conversational expert—an "architect of dialogue" to borrow a term from Harlene Anderson and Harry Goolishian (1988)—rather than an expert who is an "encyclopedia of knowledge." Clinicians do know ways to work with language so that human problems are more easily resolved. Clinicians do not, however, possess special knowledge with which they can prescribe to patients and families how they should live their lives.

Patients and families can be offered what a clinician has learned from work with other patients and families. As such, recommendations should always be presented in a tentative manner, not as context-free pronouncements of fact for patients and families to assimilate as the truth. Such statements could be variations of: "Some patients with this problem have found that meeting with the person by whom they most long to be understood is most useful. Some have found writing a letter to that person to be most useful, while others have found talking about the problem here with a friend and imagining together what a direct conversation with that person might be like is most useful. Do any of these ideas sound worth pursuing to you? Which would you want to try first? How will we tell if it has merit?" This is a "cafeteria-style" offering of ideas in which a variety of plausible avenues toward solution are laid out side by side, from which the patient and family can select (or decline to select) a path to follow (Griffith & Griffith, 1990).

Findings from scientific research studies should be made available to patients and families. However, a clinician cannot assume that probabilistic reasoning from statistical descriptions of group characteristics can provide adequate or reliable information about individual group members. It is important to deconstruct an empirical research study by describing in enough detail how the study was organized and what results were found, presenting it in such a manner that the patient and family members can collaborate in interpreting any application to their specific situation. With a family in which a daughter is suffering from anorexia nervosa, for example, statements that begin with: "Studies of patients with anorexia show . . . " should be avoided. One can, however, offer findings from the study in a form such as: "When researchers gathered 100 families with a teenage daughter with anorexia and asked each family member confidential questions about family relationships, 70% of the fathers reported that they placed little pressure on their daughters and would be pleased if they could just get well, while 75% of the daughters reported high performance pressure from their fathers and that they felt that they could never measure up to these expectations, leading the investigators to wonder whether direct conversations between fathers and daughters might bring relief to both. Does any of this sound as if it might be relevant to your situation?" Presented in this manner, the clinician joins the family in deconstructing together the epistemological process employed by the investigators, placing their findings within a specific context dictated by the limitations of their experimental methodology (Griffith & Griffith, 1990).

The patient's experience, not a scientific or societal standard, is the ultimate judge of the worth of the work between clinician and patient. Rather than stating, "It is great you are so much better. Your Hamilton Depression Scale shows that you are no longer depressed," one would ask instead, "How is the depression now compared to where we started? What things do you notice that tell you this? Your Hamilton Depression Scale Score is less than one-half of what it was when we started. Is this better or worse than your own assessment?"

The patient's and family's critique of the therapy should be sought regularly. "If there were to be anything in this therapy that would be helpful to another patient or family with a similar problem, what would that likely be? What is your understanding of how it works so that this has been helpful?"

These guidelines are social practices for organizing therapy that are alternatives to those that commonly have evolved out of biomedical science. They are ground rules for a structure within which therapeutic dialogue can spontaneously emerge. One could argue on other moral grounds that clinicians should strive to create clinical encounters with patients and families that are egalitarian to the greatest extent possible. However, the argument is made here on the basis of therapeutic efficacy. They foster emotional postures of curiosity, openness, and respect within both clinician and patients with their families. These emotional postures provide an atmosphere in which important personal narratives at the junctures of mind and body can be safely told.

TAKING INTO ACCOUNT THE IMPACT OF THE CLINICAL SETTING

Clinicians should take active responsibility for how the social structure of the clinical setting will likely influence conversations. Mind-body problems are often closely tied to fears that one would be deemed unacceptable as a person if critical life narratives were to be publicly revealed. More than with other kinds of human problems, a therapist needs to provide the most inviting setting possible when seeking to create dialogue. One would think that this point should not need to be made. For most of the past 100 years psychoanalysts have paid exquisite attention to how subtle variations in the way clinical work is structured—ground rules about when and where to meet, payment of fees, handling dual relationships between clinician and patient—can exert major effects in the outcome of the work. These concerns, usually called frame issues, are fundamental to the conduct of psychoanalytic therapies, because they affect how the transferential relationship, a vehicle of change in these therapies, evolves between clinician and patient.

An unfortunate part of the explosive growth of brief therapies during the 1970s and 1980s has been the forgetting of some valuable lessons learned by psychoanalysts in years gone by. Faced with the prospect of a dual relationship, as when a neighborhood friend requests help with a problem, many proponents of brief therapies today show no hesitancy in saying, "Now I'll take off my 'friend hat' and put on my 'therapist hat'," as if there were nothing more to it than that. The following example of a failed therapy shows how specifically problematic this can be when working with mind-body problems.

Sam Taylor was the 17-year-old son of a colleague. During the past year

Sam had developed episodic abdominal pain for which repeated tests and examinations of his gastrointestinal tract failed to show any pathology that could account for the symptoms. Sam's physician father was firmly convinced that Sam's problem was psychosomatic, related to the difficult struggle Sam was enduring in deciding on a future career and selecting an appropriate college. He sought for me (JLG) to work with his son in psychotherapy.

I questioned whether Sam could be comfortable coming to his father's colleague and workplace for therapy. However, both Sam and his father felt certain that this would not be a problem. Wishing not to offend and realizing that neither could imagine any valid reason for my hesitancy, I agreed to work with Sam.

During the first sessions, Sam talked openly about his life story. Then there came a day when he let me know that there were important things he should talk about, but he "was not ready yet." During subsequent sessions his abdominal cramping became exaggerated whenever he struggled with ambivalence over what to reveal and what to hold within himself.

We met regularly for 4 months, as I tried every maneuver I knew that might ease the way for Sam to talk. At the end of that time, when he left for college still suffering with symptoms, he acknowledged that the really important topics had not yet been broached in the therapy. He said that he finally realized that he could not talk about these things so close to home, now matter how many guarantees of confidentiality he had.

Some situations, such as that posed by Sam and his father, seem to be impossible to work out, given the constraints of the specific relationships involved. Here, my concern was not so much for the transferential relationship between Sam and myself (although a psychoanalyst might have viewed the problem through that lens). It was that Sam and I could not create a context within which authentic dialogue was possible, because the shadow of Sam's father loomed too close for Sam to talk comfortably. Had there been a good alternative clinician acceptable to both Sam and his father (often a problem in smaller communities), chances for success would have improved dramatically by referral to a more anonymous setting.

In planning a therapy, one ought to use at least the sensitivity and good sense needed to plan a successful dinner in terms of who is invited and who sits next to whom. Because of restraints imposed by the relationships involved, some dinner conversations simply cannot take place.

TAKING INTO ACCOUNT THE RELATIONAL IMPACT OF THE CLINICIAN'S EXPERT KNOWLEDGE

Clinicians should take active responsibility for the influence of their special knowledge on the therapeutic conversation. Clinicians are responsible for regulating how knowledge flows into and out of the therapy from external sources. This is not a concern about the informational content, but with the ways that possession of knowledge can shift power, subjugating some conversational participants, so that authentic dialogue is impossible. Possession of expert knowledge is toxic for dialogue when its presence in a relationship silences the voice of one of the participants.

This problem holds a heightened significance for therapy of mind-body problems, because we are often obliged to discuss problems by using physiological language (an expert language) in order to make good use of available medical treatments. Additional practical ways to couple narrative and physiological descriptions are discussed in chapter 11. The following example shows how one can minimize the shackling effects on dialogue of expert knowledge and other special, or secretly held, knowledges.

I (MEG) was called to the Children's Hospital to consult with a pediatrician eager to discharge from the hospital 9-year-old Tommy Bridges. The hacking cough that had led to Tommy's admission, however, had not improved despite intensive respiratory therapy and medical treatment. Tommy had chronic asthma, but the frequency and disabling nature of his cough were not explainable by any physiological evaluation of his relatively healthy respiratory system.

The pediatrician suspected that the magnitude of the concern and attention shown by his grandmother was providing positive reinforcement that perpetuated the cough. The pediatric nurses concurred with this suspicion and were quite frustrated that for 5 days they had been unable to observe Tommy alone. Tommy's grandmother was a constant and committed presence. "We can't even see if he coughs when she's not around, because she won't let us near him," they told me. "She wants to do all his nursing care and answers all of our questions for him."

When I first went to Tommy's hospital room, I introduced myself as a nurse clinician who worked with families of sick children. I explained that I was on the faculty of the psychiatry department and that I had a special interest in working with families who had medical illnesses, particularly when symptoms were hard to understand. She said that she had worked in her community helping families with chronically ill members, having experienced a lengthy chronic illness with her daughter. Her daughter had died several years earlier from an undiagnosed complication of her multiple sclerosis, hence Mrs. Lewis's commitment to watch over her sick grandson and be certain he get the attention he needed.

I listened to her story about the years of care she gave her daughter before the daughter died and the years of worry she spent after the death wondering whether she had been attentive enough. I eventually asked what she had learned from her experience with chronic illness and families that might be of help now with Tommy's situation. She said that she had learned that the caretakers and sick children needed to have breaks from one another from time to time. She said she needed to take a break that day. Would I stay in the room with Tommy? I could not do so at that time, but her relaxed body and her request indicated that she felt increasing comfort with me as we talked.

At the end of this meeting, I mentioned that I would make a note in the hospital chart. She immediately recoiled. I was puzzled. "What will you write in that chart about us?" she voiced with alarm, "That I am overprotective? That I am crazy?" "Not at all," I replied, "but to be sure that I am communicating what they need to understand, would you help me write the note?" I brought the chart from the nurses' station, and she worked with me to construct the note. She felt that we should record her story, so that the staff could realize that this hospitalization was especially stressful to her because of her experience with her daughter who died, but that the staff could also know that she also brought extra nursing expertise from that same experience. I met back with Tommy alone the next day as his grandmother had requested. As the nurses appreciated her personal story, she decided she could take the breaks she needed and leave Tommy alone with them.

Based on this understanding of language, stories, and social processes, one would not be surprised that the sequestering of knowledge within hospital charts and private conversations among professionals had such a pronounced impact on the therapeutic relationship with Tommy's grandmother. In its biological sense, language exists as a reciprocal signaling through which human mammals coordinate their bodily states, like ships holding formation through the back-and-forth flashing of semaphore flags. Every conversation defines a community. A person excluded from this signaling not only loses access to information but also loses a biological, psychological, and spiritual sense of community with other humans. Such a person loses the ability to touch other humans and to be touched.

Scientific biomedical culture is organized by implicit rules about knowledge that render it problematic for the citizens it is supposed to serve. The epistemological standard for medical science consists of consensus opinions by the "scientific community"—medical school faculty, medical journal audiences, medical societies. Only those who can speak the language of science can be members of this community. Only those human experiences that are validated by the scientific community as "real" can be discussed in this scientific discourse.

Tommy's grandmother could not participate as a member of the scientific community for a variety of reasons. She could not speak the languages of medical science. The personal experiences that held her greatest attention would be considered by medical science to hold little validity as relevant information for Tommy's problem. The important conversations among members of the scientific medical community occurred in places where she had no access—medical charts, coffee room discussions, clinical case conferences, professional meetings. In addition to her exclusion by the medical community, she also felt emotionally excluded by the nurses. Although she might otherwise have felt a ready kinship with them, as she had worked as a private-duty nurse in her local community, she had felt alienated from the hospital nurses, as if they were extensions of the physicians. This was understandable when I saw that the nursing orders were for them to count how many times Tommy coughed in a 15-minute period and to compare that with the number of times his grandmother reported. It was also requested that the nurses try to "get Tommy alone" apart from his grandmother to determine whether the coughing occurred in her absence.

Tommy's grandmother's position in the medical social structure was that of an untouchable—invisible, untouching and untouched, yet dependent on this medical society for sustenance. But so long as the important communications regarding Tommy took place in private conversations among medical professionals and in written communications shared in the hospital chart, the voice of the grandmother was excluded from a conversation that would determine her grandchild's medical fate. She could choose whether to accept this position of subjugation or to fend off any relationship with the medical system that would bind her. Small wonder that she had chosen the latter course.

Specific actions were taken that enabled the grandmother to enter into language and into community with her clinicians. She thus became a member of the community of "standard observers" entrusted with specifying what is valid knowledge. This change in social status was reflected in the dramatic opening of new possibilities for a therapeutic relationship between clinician and family.

In other cases, it has been important to refuse participation in social practices whose effect is to place the clinician in a role of holder of secret information. Often, medical records or a hospital chart accompanies the patient to the referral. Usually, these records are documents describing stories about the problem that have never been made available to the patient for correction or expansion. It is wise to refrain from reviewing such records, other than accessing the necessary medical (physiological) information, until such time that they can be reviewed collaboratively with the patient, requesting comments as to any errors or omissions. It is often customary for a referring clinician to initiate a referral by relating to the consultant clinician his or her version of the story of the problem. When possible, it is more useful to avoid such information, tactfully telling the referring clinician that his or her description is needed, but that it is preferable to meet the patient or family first with no prior information.

It is best, of course, for the referring physician to participate in the initial conversation with the patient or family, so that the discussion of the purpose of the consultation, its backgrounds, and the physician's thought about solutions can be conducted in the family's presence. When this cannot be arranged, whatever information that has been transmitted from the referring physician can be fully related to the patient in the first meeting. The patient and family members can then make any corrections or additions needed, so that there is a mutual understanding of the problem before the work begins. Patients are assured that they will be party to any significant conversations with other clinicians regarding their care. Patients are sent copies of any written communications with other clinicians. Their aid, in fact, is often obtained in composing reports, letters, and other written documents that are necessary during the course of therapy. This requires that the clinician discipline himself or herself to use the same language in conversations with other clinicians and in the clinician's own private musings that the clinician uses in conversing in sessions with the patient and family—language that accurately describes everything witnessed in the therapy session, yet also would be found affiliative by family members if they were to hear it or read it. These practices run counter to common habits of language use in most clinical settings, which can be described as "what the patient and family don't hear doesn't hurt them."

This approach to therapy offers a bonus. It generally does not hinder, and can even help, the therapy when the patient and family members read their medical chart, view communications between clinician and other professionals, or even sit in on a formal presentation about their case among a group of clinicians. As a clinician, it is much more relaxing not to feel obligated to sequester information.

Using Language to Construct a Conversational Domain for Talking about Personal Stories

Mind-body problems that have been resistant to repeated efforts by clinicians to treat them are more often than not immersed in monological conversations between clinician, patient, and family members. These "dueling monologues" are repetitive, sequential speeches, protests, justifications, and arguments by each of those involved in the problem, but little mutual listening or understanding is taking place. Creating conditions that favor dialogue, not monologue, seems to be essential to the therapy of mind-body problems.

The tailoring of language for a specific therapy is termed the developing of a conversational domain, as described in conversation theory (Braten, 1987; Pask, 1976). A conversational domain is present when all the conversational participants have engaged in a process of speaking, listening, and reflecting, from which has arisen a mutually negotiated, specific language for talking about the problem of the therapy and its needed solution. Its formation closely resembles the growth of understanding between participants in a game of charades, where the team is limited to pantomime and gesture in its communications. The team gestures to the other team, receiving stumbling words or phrases as signals for whether understanding had been achieved. In the back-and-forth gesturing and signaling, words are finally produced that match the intent of the gesturing team, and excited nodding by the participants marks the correct response. As in charades, the mutual signaling by participants in a conversation when specific metaphors and idioms are used alerts us that understanding has occurred and a conversational domain has been opened.

The notion of a conversational domain arose during the 1970s among cognitive scientists who strove to understand how an organism could preserve its identity as an autonomous entity yet be changed through communicative interactions with other autonomous entities (Varela, 1979). Gordon Pask (1976), an iconoclastic English educator, created conversation theory as a framework for understanding how humans and "intelligent" machines could communicate. Carried into human engagements through language, this idea provides a useful tool for understanding how some conversations fail and others succeed among clinicians, patients, and families.

The creation of a conversational domain is closely related to a shift from monologues to dialogues in conversation. The Norwegian sociologist Stein Braten (1987) has usefully pointed out the interrelationships between dialogue, monologue, and creativity (or lack of it). Simply put, creative ideas most often spring out of dialogical, not monological, conversations. Braten means dialogue in the sense of Martin Buber and Fyodor Dostoevski, as a respectful reflection on multiple perspectives that stand side by side within the same conversation. Out of this speaking, listening, reflecting, a crisscrossing of perspectives arises within which new ideas are born. By contrast, monologues are characterized by a single dominant perspective, regardless how many persons are present in the conversation. By this definition, Socrates' conversation with the little slave boy who rediscovered the Pythagorean theorem was a Socratic monologue, not a Socratic dialogue as it has been called.

· We can perhaps best understand what a conversational domain is by examining efforts to talk about mind-body problems when that domain is absent. For example, In *Hannah and Her Sisters,* a sketch called "The Hypochondriac" shows Woody Allen, as a television producer, Nick, complaining of stomach pain amidst the maddening pace of his Manhattan lifestyle as he begs Tagamets off his friends. Nick goes to his internist seeking reassurance, mentioning as an aside that he has had some hearing loss in his right ear ("Or is it my left ear?"). His doctor reassures him that "it is nothing." Yet, he wants to have Nick tested to rule out the one-in-a-million possibility that he has a brain tumor.

At the hospital, Nick's care is turned over to a specialist who pursues the tumor possibility relentlessly with audiograms, tomograms, and CT scans. Nick hyperventilates with anxiety. We hear the words of the specialist conversing with Nick: "I wasn't too happy with the results of your EMG, or your BSER either, which is why I sent you to tomography, which is all that stuff you saw rolling around." He tries to be helpful to Nick by showing Nick the actual X-rays: "That gray area is what I hoped we wouldn't run into."

But along a separate soundtrack we also hear Nick's inner conversation with himself: "Okay. Take it easy. He didn't say you had anything. He just doesn't like the spot on your X-ray. That's all. It doesn't mean you have anything. Don't jump to conclusions." But his terror builds and builds until he is shouting to himself, "I'm dying! I'm dying! . . . There's a tumor inside my head that is the size of a basketball!" He begins feeling all sorts of other new bodily sensations that validate his certainty of impending doom. The intensity continues to escalate, until predictably the specialist walks in and announces, "Well, you are just fine. There is nothing here at all."

At first Nick is elated, but then he stops to think, "I'm not going to go today. I'm okay. I'm not going to go tomorrow. . . . But, eventually, I am going to be in that position!" His bodily vigilance returns, and he feels so depressed that he begins thinking about suicide.

We can see how the encounters between Nick and the medical professionals were essentially parallel monologues, with Nick's evolving private narrative that defined his selfhood pushed out of the clinician-patient conversations. The clinicians undoubtedly felt that an adequate dialogue with sufficient explanations and reassurances had occurred. But Nick heard the implicit request to submit and responded by listening quietly, attempting to accept the domination of his experience by medical science. His overt behavior was submissive to the medical specialists, but his body felt no better; his private dialogue had not been banished by the medical-expert discourse but went underground, revealing itself only in his private thoughts and maintaining unabated, exclusive control of his bodily experience. The clinicians showed no curiosity about Nick's personal experience or his personal vocabulary of that experience. There was no effort by the clinicians to co-construct with Nick a conversational domain within which Nick's experience—and his body—could find a voice.

Like Nick's physician, one can move through many, perhaps most, of life's interactions by using a functional language made up of only the shells of words. Through silencing one's bodily expressions, conversations can proceed in which ideas flow quickly and discussions are finished without waiting for the bodies' responses to catch up or express an opinion. Using these husks of words, one can talk with one's head, unslowed by the pace of one's heart. Nick's medical specialist is expert in the use of such language that within limits is adequate for moving, manipulating, and organizing others in directions he wishes them to go. The price paid for this efficiency, though, is the loss of a language through which Nick's body can speak and listen. If, instead, a conversational domain is created for dialogue in therapy, the language is rebuilt so that it is again suitable for the body.

In addition to the care shown in structuring a therapeutic conversation, two additional strategies are helpful in building a conversational domain: using the patient's language and following body language.

USING THE PATIENT'S UNIQUE LANGUAGE AS THE BASIS FOR THE THERAPY

The best first step toward building a conversational domain is to notice attentively the patient's own language for talking about the problem, then building on this unique vocabulary of personal experience to create a language that is idiosyncratic for this specific therapy.

For many years masterful teachers of psychotherapy, from Harry Stack Sullivan to George Kelly and Harry Goolishian (Goolishian & Winderman, 1988), have directed their students to begin therapy by "learning the language of the patient" (Kelly, 1963, p. 174). For most students, this instruction has initially seemed counterintuitive, because it is out of step with a commonly held perspective on scientific expertise that would begin by training the patient to adopt the scientific language and worldview the clinician brings. However, our discussion of language provides good reasons why there is more therapeutic power in working within the specific language the patient brings. We are seeking a relationship organized around emotional postures of curiosity, openness, and respect; we will likely not find such a relationship if our first step is a request that the patient submit to an external authority by leaving behind the language in which the patient is in dialogue with his or her body. We are primarily concerned that the language of the therapy resonate with bodily processes that the patient describes. Specific, idiosyncratic language that the patient initially brings is far more likely to provide this resonance than a generic brand of talk that is so broadly defined that anyone in the culture understands it.

We can illustrate this process in therapy through examining more closely the therapy of Mrs. Merton, who was referred by her internist for treatment of her unremitting headaches. In her initial interviews, she told, bit by bit, the story of her yearning to be an artist, the stigma attached to art in her family because of her "black sheep" uncle who was a depressed artist with a violent temper, and the emptiness of her present work as an accountant.

Mrs. Merton told how she was very successful, but unhappy, in her job as an accountant. Through college she had been a gifted artist. In her family mythology, however, art had a dark side, inextricably linked to mental illness because of the stories about a great-uncle who was a renowned artist but also frequently psychotic and violent. In her last year of college, she switched her major studies from fine arts to accounting, following in her father's footsteps.

Recently, however, she found that her artistic side had reawakened through her experience of parenting her young daughter. She wanted to deemphasize her professional work in her life in order to spend more time at home with her daughter but felt that her parents could only accept her within her persona of successful businesswoman. Her debilitating headaches and nausea settled the issue, forcing her to sharply reduce her hours on the job.

Mrs. Merton raged against her headaches. She experienced them as an external evil force that she should be expected to resist through willpower. Her inner voice admonished, "Stop this right now. You should be back at work," and "You are being weak." She hid her inner dilemma from her husband, whom she did not wish to burden in his new job. She also did not discuss it with her parents, who saw her symptoms as indicating spiritual weakness and a need to reinvolve her life in her church.

In the initial session, I (JLG) had noted her root metaphors in the language with which she talked about her life with headaches—"weakness," "crazy," "artistic," and "success." As she told the saga of her illness from the beginning, I inquired about critical parts of her life story that gave definition to each of these metaphors, permitting her to talk uninterrupted until she had finished her story. I continued to search for the exact meanings of words as she used them, until she nodded her approval.

During the therapy, each metaphor was treated as if it were a label on a file drawer filled with life stories—stories of "artistic," stories of "weakness," stories of "crazy." Only as these stories were told did we come to a common understanding of the meaning of her words.

We talked at length about her dilemma, examining each of its sides and seeking a precise understanding of its terms, while refraining from forcing a resolution within the session. By her third visit, however, she, without prompting from me, had limited her contact with her parents, had begun talking openly with her husband, and had acted on a clear choice to direct her primary attention away from work to her child, with whom she now found the place of her artistic expression in her parenting. The headaches improved until they could be managed with minimal medication.

One can recognize critical language of experience when a patient uses particular words, phrases, or idiosyncratic expressions repeatedly to describe his or her experience. The body shows markers for important language—a change in tone of voice, facial expression, state of muscle tension, breathing, or posture when particular words or phrases are spoken. Persons often introduce their metaphors with the expression, "It is like . . . ," or "It makes me feel like . . . " When a particular metaphor or expression is noted, a clinician appropriately can respond with his or her own metaphor ("Is it like . . . ?") to learn to what extent the different images of the world match. It is in this back-and-forth exchanging of metaphors, in the speaking, listening, and reflecting, that a conversational domain takes shape. The assumption of understanding can only be tentative. Only a speaker can say whether he or she was understood in a given moment. The expression, "I understand," is best avoided by a clinician who genuinely strives for understanding.

One never knows for sure how far understanding extends. We only know for sure the occasions when understanding breaks down. One of our clearest recollections of breakdown in understanding took place outside any professional setting. While traveling in Denmark, our children yearned for some good, greasy American food. Our 7-year-old son begged us to locate a grilled cheese sandwich. In a Copenhagen street market, we found an elderly woman selling the open-faced sandwiches for which Scandanavia is famous. I tried to pantomime the making of a grilled cheese sandwich while saying "smor-brod" (my best approximation) and "cheese-toast" alternatively. The old woman, speaking no English, made the same motions in response, nodding and saying "smor-brod, cheese-toast." As we nodded enthusiastically to one another, our son, watching, relaxed with relief. The woman disappeared. Returning a moment later, she produced, with a broad smile, a piece of black bread stacked with white cheese, a tomato slice, and a radish on top. After one glance at the sandwich, it was clear that the parents, not the children, would be eating this "grilled cheese."

The Danish woman and our family had each exchanged enough gestures, in body and in speech, to establish mutual understanding. There was no reason to suspect any lack of understanding . . . until the sandwich appeared. We can never know that we understand another person. We can only know the fractures that appear, the breakdowns in understanding. Although there is little surprise in seeing such breakdowns occurring between two persons from alien cultures, we often fail to realize how equally wide gulfs in understanding regularly appear between two persons within the same culture using the same words from the same language.

One is wise, then, never to assume that a clinician's innocent paraphrase of a patient's language in fact achieves understanding of the language. One remains on safest ground when the therapy is built around a person's exact use of language, repeatedly returning throughout the therapy to the patient's own words.

Many approaches to therapy encourage a clinician to begin by showing a credulous attitude in order to gain the patient's confidence, after which an indoctrination into the clinician's language and worldview can subtly begin. Our proposal is a more radical alternative in asking that the clinician dare to accept the patient's language on its own terms, without further interpretation.

One can never assume preknowledge about words and their meanings that participants hold upon entering a conversation, nor is it sufficient to use a dictionary to referee the meanings. Specific meanings of words in a conversational domain are anchored in specific stories of lived experience that belong solely to the speaker, until the stories themselves are shared in conversation with others.

GUIDING CONVERSATIONS BY WATCHING AND FOLLOWING THE BODIES OF PARTICIPANTS

To solve problems, one may need to talk about topics that are frightening, shameful, or enraging to the patient or family members. A clinician must learn how to enable discussion of such topics to proceed, while also enabling conversational participants to remain within emotional postures of tranquility. A competent clinician, therefore, needs perceptual skills that can guide an approach to the boundary of patients' and family members' umwelts, without trangressing them and thus triggering alarm. This "walking the edge of the umwelt" is a good definition for pacing a therapy.

Skill in pacing consists of learning to detect subtle signs that the clinician, in bringing up certain topics of conversation or pressing for answers to questions, or deciding to continue a discussion a bit longer, has moved into a liminal zone where, notwithstanding continuing social courtesies by the patient or family members, definite signs of alarm have appeared, presaging flight or fight should the clinician persist. These signs of alarm are expressed in shifts of body state among conversational participants—a change to rapid or shallow breathing, closed-off or rigid body postures, tight lips, frequent swallowing, tightness or loudness of voice, hesitation during speech, aggressive or "walling-off" gestures, a tentative handshake, choosing to sit at the periphery of the group, a drifting or averted gaze. These signs, when detected, mean that the clinician should slow down the pace of the session or at least inquire respectfully about the comfort level of the session participants.

For example, Alex Gates, a 15-year-old boy, had been referred with his family to our family therapy clinic, because he had missed so many days of school because of various physical symptoms that it had become questionable whether he could be promoted to the next grade. The first session proceeded smoothly. The family connected warmly to the psychiatry resident as she elicited their stories about the problem. After the first session, Alex went to school 4 days that week, an unusual achievement for him.

The second session focused on ways to build on this success. However, he then missed 4 days the next week because of stomachaches. Frustrated with her own actions, the resident related the events of the third session to me (MEG). She was concerned that the family had not taken Alex to his family physician until the end of the week in order to find out whether this was a problem that required medical treatment or whether he should have been encouraged to go on to school despite his discomfort. As she asked questions about their actions, she noted that Alex sat silent with arms folded. She suggested that they sign a release of information so that she could communicate freely with the doctor in devising a plan so that any time Alex showed illness, he could obtain an immediate medical evaluation in order to learn whether he should go on to school. The family members, including Alex, signed the consent form. However, when the resident asked at the end of the session about a return appointment, Alex said, "We aren't going to come back. You are doing the same thing the other doctors did." The resident said, "The thing was, I knew that he was going to say that. I knew it when I first walked out of the room to get the consent form, but I didn't know how to stop it. We were following the plan we had agreed to last week."

The resident's plan for involving the family physician in a comprehensive treatment plan for Alex was conceptually sound. However, following the plan left her unable to attend to Alex's bodily signals, so that she and he no longer were in a conversational domain.

Metaphorically, one can think of this careful modulation of language through following bodily signs as building a linguistic dwelling within which discourse about threatening or painful topics can be safely conducted. Understanding thus can be viewed as a biological phenomenon whose boundaries are marked by the bodily signals of the conversational participants.

Engaging Oneself in the Conversation to Open Access to Knowledge

Each emotional body posture dictates an epistemological stance that acts as a window through which certain descriptions of the world can enter as knowledge, but other descriptions cannot (Griffith & Griffith, 1992a). This window delimits the world as it can be experienced. It is important that a clinician take responsibility for his or her epistemological stance in therapy.

Sometimes, the emotional postures of participants in a conversation couple, so that each participant prompts a repetitive emergence of the complementary emotional posture from the other. When this coupling of emotions occurs, as in the coemergence of joyful-merging/joyful-merging between two lovers, or coupling of attacking/appeasing in an abusive relationship, or coupling of instructing/learning from in a pedagogical relationship, whatever reality can be experienced has been already preselected by these coupled emotional postures. In a human relationship, a coupling of emotional postures is destiny for its epistemology.

One can see, then, why attention to the coupling of emotional postures is so important in a developing relationship between clinician and patient. From the patient's perspective, the clinician can be transformed into a facilitative, paternalistic, supportive, or sadistic kind of person, depending on the coupling of emotion within which the relationship grows. For any of these descriptions, the patient can point to specific actions by the clinician that can seem to justify the perception. From a clinician's perspective, the same patient, depending on the coupling of emotions, can be found to be helpless and pitiable, manipulative and controlling, or competent and wise. Like a multifaceted diamond, the patient and clinician each show a different shade and color depending on the emotional light of the relationship (Griffith, Griffith, & Slovik, 1990).

The sticking point for therapeutic work with mind-body problems, as seen with Mr. O'Malley and Mr. Duquesnay in chapter 1, is the frequency and manner in which treatment relationships have tended to abort in their early stages, with harmful consequences for both patient and clinician. In what ways, then, might an understanding of emotional posture, coupling of emotions, and epistemological stance build for us a vessel that can navigate an often treacherous passage to a therapeutic relationship?

In our clinical work, we have traveled simultaneously in two different directions with these ideas. One direction, not discussed until chapter 11, enters the physiological domain. There, the concept of emotional posture provides a clinician with a point where physiological and psychological descriptions of behavior can meet. Physiologically, shifts between emotional postures of tranquility and mobilization are regulated to a great extent by several simply organized, primitive neuronal systems located within mammalian brains in the upper brainstem and the base of the two cerebral hemispheres. Although our understanding of these systems is rudimentary at best, we do know enough to outline a way to use medications to bias the functioning of these systems to favor emotional postures of tranquility. The other direction, discussed in this chapter, is to find ways of accomplishing the same thing using language.

Selecting Emotional Postures

Building a conversational domain for dialogue is easier when a clinician resides in the same neighborhood of bodily experience as the patient's and family members'. There are two tried-and-true methods through which a clinician can select an emotional posture with which to enter the therapeutic conversation, physiological tracking and careful choice of therapy assumptions.

PHYSIOLOGICAL TRACKING AND MIRRORING

A clinician can mirror the breathing, posture, and bodily movements of patients and family members as a way of opening a window into their experiential world.

For example, a young woman, Christy, asked that I (MEG) help her to "win over or get past" a man. Being an athlete, she had requested that I be a "psychological coach," because her own efforts had failed. "It's like I'm working against myself. I'm getting weaker, and I feel like a wimp." In her daily life, she actually was neglecting her workouts and feeling weaker and energyless.

I attempted to be a good coach by helping her to strategize how to use her many personal strengths in this relationship. However, we agreed after a few weeks that we were getting nowhere. Christy was disgusted with herself and blamed herself that I could not better understand her, just as she blamed herself that her boyfriend could not understand her.

In desperation one day I decided perhaps I was listening to the lyrics but not to the music that Christy was conveying to me. I listened as if she were speaking French, a language that I do not speak. Instead of listening so much to her words, I tried to place myself in the bodily configuration in which she sat—with rapid and shallow breathing, stiffly leaning forward with a tense body, arms held tight and immobile on the chair. From this position, I listened.

She spoke logically, calmly, with flat intonation about spying on her fiancé who had been with another woman. She told how she was embarrassed to have stooped to spying but was relieved to know the truth about his recent strange behavior. It was clear to her that she should stop "wasting her life" on him and that his lying and cheating were old patterns that would not change. "My friends have been telling me for years that I deserve better. I've known what he was doing all along, but I couldn't make myself leave him. I don't know why. I'm sure you agree with my friends, but how can I make myself do it?"

On listening this time, however, I was aware of more than the progression of ideas in her words. I was distracted by an awful sensation in my throat, like the bad taste of acid after gagging. With uncertainty, I told her my experience of her words, "Christy, as I've been sitting here I've been having this strange feeling, like I'm going to gag or vomit, though I know I'm not. I wondered if this story ever brings these kinds of feelings to you?"

Surprised, she looked straight into my eyes. "That's it! That's exactly how I feel. I want to throw up, but I can't. I feel that way a lot . . . I can't throw up, and I can't eat." She began to cry. "But how did you know?"

"I didn't know," I said, not wishing to appear magical. "I just knew how I felt as I listened and wondered if there was a connection."

"There's a connection. . . . This is the first time I have felt you understood." She wept freely with relief.

We went on to talk about the awful feeling of not being able to throw up or eat. She remembered times when she had felt that way as a child and was finally able to experience a gentle sympathy for herself that eased the self-contempt she held.

In recommending these techniques, we take sharp exception to efforts to use mirroring and matching techniques for manipulating behavior. Some hypnotists have prided themselves in their successes in eliciting a particular behavior from a person outside the person's conscious awareness. In recent years there also has been an attempt (neurolinguistic programming) to create a behavioral technology out of the hypnotist Milton Erickson's work (Bandler & Grinder, 1982), through which one could, without awareness of the other, manipulate sex from a lover or a raise from one's boss (Gottlieb, 1992). Employed in this manner, neurolinguistic programming differs, because it works from emotional postures of managing, controlling, and deceiving. In our work, we seek synchronization of bodies as a way to enter the experiential world of the patient, not a way to predict or control the patient's behavior.

CHOOSING TREATMENT ASSUMPTIONS CAREFULLY

Clinicians can select those particular assumptions about the patient, the therapeutic process, the problem and its needed solution that will create emotional postures of curiosity, openness, and respect within the clinician. The main influence clinicians have over the coupling of emotions during therapy lies in how they can control the emotional postures with which they themselves enter the relationship. A clinician can disable a destructive coupling of emotion by declining to offer back to the patient the kind of emotional posture anticipated among "normal" human responses. For example, a clinician encountering a patient who is on guard, apparently withholding information, might naturally assume that there is something important to be hidden that must be ferreted out by interrogation. But for the clinician to enter the relationship with an emotional posture of suspicion befitting interrogation will likely turn the patient's fear into flight. The clinician, however, can enter the interaction with an emotional posture of respect and acceptance if he or she assumes, first, that building a relationship is more important than gathering information, and, second, that the patient may hold a valid understanding of the problem in which there is indeed wisdom in self-disclosing only with caution. As another example, a clinician encountering a patient whose complaints of physical suffering appear out of proportion to the medical evidence of disease easily feels manipulated or exploited, which invites an emotional posture of scorn toward the patient. But the clinician can remain in an emotional posture of respect if he or she chooses to assume that the patient is blocked by as yet unnamed agents or forces from communicating distress in another manner.

Similarly, a clinician can nurture the growth of a new, more desirable coupling of emotions by offering consistently to a patient emotional postures that invite reciprocal postures the clinician seeks. Although a desired atmosphere of curiosity, openness, and respect is a cocreation of both participants in a therapeutic dialogue, it is one of the specific responsibilities of the clinician to enter the therapy room within emotional postures that invite this evolution of relationship.

Toward this end, a clinician can choose the basic assumptions with which he or she will interpret his or her experience of the therapy (Griffith & Griffith, 1992a). Many of the assumptions we value either are simple truths or have been stated by others before us.

1.) Patients and family members as human beings share more similarities than differences with the clinician. A readiness to see similarities in personhood augments the building of a positive relationship, but a readiness to see differences augments a diagnostic scrutiny that classifies the other as an object. A therapist can use the knowledge of his or her personal experiences as a preknowledge to understanding the other only to the extent to which he or she is ready to see similarities instead of differences.

2.) Family members are ordinary people leading everyday lives who unfortunately have encountered unusual and difficult life circumstances (White & Epston, 1990). This assumption runs counter to psychopathological assumptions broadly held in Western culture, in which the problems of the "mentally ill" are considered to be reducible to intrapsychic mental processes or to abnormal brain physiology. However, a readiness to see problems as existing *between* persons in language, social practices, and institutions, rather than *within* their persons, biases the therapist toward respectful ways of experiencing that patient and family members.

3.) When a person or a family with a problem requests psychotherapy, it is because they are struggling with a dilemma for which the kind of conversation needed for its resolution cannot occur. An expectancy for discovering hidden constraints that bind persons and families to their suffering prepares a curiosity for hearing their stories in a therapeutic manner.

4.) Persons and families always possess more lived experience than is contained in the available narratives about their problem. As the anthropologist Clifford Geertz (1986) has pointed out, there is always a surplus of lived experience available for understanding one's life. When the clinician maintains confidence that this unseen resource is ready at hand when needed, he or she is likely to notice unused resources among the life experiences of patients and family members and to be curious about how they might be employed.

5.) Persons and family members in their deepest desires do not wish to harm themselves or others. Long-hidden yearnings to show and receive love are likely to disclose themselves only to the eyes of a therapist who already believes in the possibility of their presence.

6.) A clinician cannot understand the meaning of the language a person uses until they have talked together about it. Approaching dialogue from a position of "not knowing," as Anderson and Goolishian (1992) have emphasized, is essential if one is to work with meanings that are locally determined within the therapy dialogue.

7.) Change is always possible. The converse, a belief that change cannot occur, precludes openness.

8.) A person or a family with a problem wishes to be free of the problem. The converse, a belief that patient and family members "want to be sick" or "need to be sick," precludes respect.

9.) A clinician cannot know for sure what actions family members need to take for the problem to resolve. The converse, a sense of certainty by the therapist about what does and does not need to happen, precludes curiosity.

Many before us have of course valued some of these assumptions as ethical injunctions to which a good therapist should submit himself or herself. But this opening up of a new experiential world does not take place when one attempts to impose these principles on oneself as ethical injunctions. Defining a statement as an ethical injunction presumes in the first place that a flawed reality exists, in which the ethical behavior would not naturally occur. With courage and forbearance, one can live in that world as it should be but is not. Although this is an honorable striving, living turns into toil, and the striving breaks down under stress.

We advocate these assumptions for a different reason. When a clinician selects one of these statements as a reality assumption, his or her emotional posture tends to reconfigure, prejudicing how the clinician experiences the patient and family and their problem. In this way, one literally can choose a world whose atmosphere is one of openness, curiosity, and respect—perceptions, thoughts, and behaviors that best live in that atmosphere then follow. *Selecting the reality*, rather than *enforcing the action*, is the more therapeutic path to follow.

A clinician working with patients who present mind-body problems must nurture an interest in how one's emotion, cognition, and epistemology facilitate or hinder discovery of the kind of knowledge needed to resolve the problems. Knowledge is effective action; emotion is a bodily readiness for action (Maturana & Varela, 1987). We see, then, how the wisdom of the body is housed in its emotional postures.

As clinicians, our competence lies in finding ways to style the dance of emotional postures between clinician, patient, and family members, so that it favors discovery of the kind of knowledge that we anticipate will be needed if the problem of the therapy is to resolve. So, we ask:

- What kind of knowledge might possibly be needed to solve the problem?
- What epistemological stance would maximize the likelihood of discovering this needed knowledge?
- Which emotional postures would embody this epistemological stance?
- How can the coupling of emotions between myself as clinician and the patient and family members shift so as to evoke these needed emotional postures?
- As clinician, how can I select an emotional posture that will prompt this shift in coupling of emotions?
- What changes in my assumptions about the patient, family, problem, or needed solution will facilitate the desired reconfiguring of my own emotional posture?

This is the challenge of therapy.

CHAPTER 5

A Telling That Heals

*A genuine conversation gives me access to thoughts that I did not
know myself capable of, that I was not capable of.*
                                   —Maurice Merleau-Ponty

"**W**ANT TO SEE some pseudoseizures?" my neurologist colleague
spoke to me (JLG) on the elevator. "Go see Mr. Duquesnay in room 511. He's
got the worst I have ever seen."

Mr. Jimmy Duquesnay was a 45-year-old man who had been treated in
the epilepsy clinic for 2 years. His seizures had been occurring more and
more frequently over the past 6 months, despite careful adjustments of his
anticonvulsant medications, including trials of new medications. Finally, he
had been admitted to the hospital, because the avenues available for out-
patient treatment had been exhausted.

In the hospital, as his physicians watched in frustration, he continued to
have daily seizures. The form of the seizures was suspect, however: The pattern of jerking and the shifts in his conscious awareness did not fit those
expected with epileptic seizures. Finally, a split-screen EEG study was conducted, in which a videotape of his seizure behavior was superimposed
above a record of his electrical brain waves. His seizure behavior was occurring despite his normal EEG. The diagnosis was confirmed—nonepileptic
seizures, or pseudoseizures.

Unfortunately, the neurologist's report angered his wife, and Mr.
Duquesnay's seizures in fact escalated on hearing the news about the normal
EEG. His seizures had become so violent that, by the time I met him, he was
physically restrained in bed with his arms and legs strapped down with
leather binds in order to prevent him from harming himself with his violent
thrashing. Our psychiatric consultation team had been called for assistance
but could offer little to diminish his symptoms.

The treating neurologist tried to confront him tactfully with the evidence that he had a psychiatric, not a neurological problem. The consulting psychiatrist could see no opening through which psychotherapy could be attempted and had begun administering tranquilizing medications. By the time I met Mr. Duquesnay, proceedings had been initiated for chronic hospitalization at a state psychiatric facility.

Mr. Duquesnay was a sandy-haired, middle-aged man who most of his life had fished for shrimp off the Gulf Coast. Because of his seizures, his doctors several years earlier had raised concerns about his sailing his own boat, so he sold the boat to his brother. Now, he mostly helped out the shrimp fleet with work on shore.

Mr. Duquesnay arrived at the interview room in a wheelchair, accompanied by his wife and teenage son, Pierre. They entered silently, offering only the ritual smiles and nods to my hello. I explained the structure of the interview, that I would be talking with them while Melissa would be watching and listening, then later offering her thoughts. She shook hands with each family member and retired to the observation room. I began by requesting that only those topics be discussed that could be discussed within emotional postures of tranquility:

JLG: I will ask any question that I feel it might be useful to ask. But if a question feels intrusive or inappropriate to discuss at this time, just say that you wish to "pass" on that question. I will go on to another question. I think that we only need to discuss today those things that can comfortably be discussed. I understand that every family has some private matters that would be inappropriate for discussion in a setting such as this.

The family members each nodded in assent. Mrs. Duquesnay smiled in a friendly manner, but Mr. Duquesnay sat silently in his wheelchair, tremulous, brow furrowed, looking frightened and confused. He seemed much older than his age of 45. His son and wife were quick to help him, anticipating his needs.

JLG: [Leaning forward] To begin with, tell me what you think I would need to know about your problem in order to understand it? I've read your chart, and there is a lot of information there, but, from your perspective, what is the story of your illness? Where would you start if you were to tell me about it in a way so I would understand it?

Mr. Duquesnay stared at me, his eyes never deviating, even when there were distracting noises or motions. He looked self-effacing and apologetic but also guarded. I listened quietly with my chin propped on my fist. I listened closely for the metaphors and stories they would choose for telling me about the illness.

MR. DUQUESNAY: I was driving a pickup truck coming from Leakesville. I was driving home with a friend driving behind me. That is all I remember. The next thing I knew, I was in the hospital. They said my truck was pulled over on the side of the road. My foot was on the brake, and I was laid over on the side of the seat. That is all I remember.

The family had come to the session under a cloud of humiliation, feeling blamed for their husband's and father's failure to respond to treatment. The first task—and perhaps only task—of this interview would be to help Mr. Duquesnay and his family to shift from emotional postures of mobilization to those of tranquility. The only tool that could be employed would be the careful use of language.

In planning the session, I avoided situations that could obstruct the building of a conversational domain, particularly my possessing information to which the patient and family were not privy. I sought only that information that was essential for understanding the physiological parameters of the problem, his EEG and magnetic resonance imaging (MRI) scan reports, findings on neurological examinations, a list of medications administered. I chose not to read, prior to meeting the family, descriptions and speculations from other involved clinicians that were written in his hospital chart. I wanted to organize this session around their personal accounts of the problem.

The selection of participants in the interview was not ideal. It would have been better to meet with the entire group of people who were engaged around the problem. This grouping, the problem-organized system, would have included the neurologists treating Mr. Duquesnay. Because the physician-patient relationship here appeared to be near an irreversible termination, we did not press for them to meet together. It was important, however, that the family—not Mr. Duquesnay as an individual—be present.

MRS. DUQUESNAY: He went into a hospital. They had a neurologist there. His mother spent the night with him, so I could go home and rest. While she was sleeping on her cot, his mother heard something fall. Jimmy had gotten up to go to the bathroom. She asked him if he needed some help, and he said, "No." Then she heard him hit the floor. She called Dr. Stanton who saw that Jimmy was having a seizure, a grand mal seizure. That was the first one. Ever since then, it has never stopped. . . .
JLG: When you say "never stopped," do mean every day? Or occasionally?

By keeping the dialogue of the session close to specific language used by the family and by asking questions that make finer and finer distinctions, a conversational domain began to form within which the interview could be conducted.

MRS. DUQUESNAY: He did have seizures every day for a long, long time. I kept a record. Every time he had one, I wrote down how many he had, what time, and all this stuff.

JLG: How many would there be?

MRS. DUQUESNAY: [Sitting up and leaning forward for emphasis] He's had seven, eight, or nine at a time! . . . Or he would have one, and that would be it. Unfortunately, there has been no pattern. It is odd, really. We'll be sitting there, and he'll say, "Jackie, I feel weird." I'll say, "What do you mean, baby?" He'll say, "I just feel weird." There would be something strange about his expression . . . like he was out in space.

MR. DUQUESNAY: A blank stare.

MRS. DUQUESNAY: Maybe it doesn't happen right then. . . . Sometimes you can call him back, "Jimmy! Jimmy! Jimmy!" But it won't last, and he goes right back into it. That is why at night I won't even try to make him come out of it, because in the past I have sat up all night doing it. As long as I would pat him and try to get him out of it, he would be all right. . . .

[I paused for Mr. Duquesnay to move from his wheelchair to the sofa, while Mrs. Duquesnay curled up, relaxing, at the other end.]

JLG: What would be your main sense about what needs to be done with the way things are right now? If I were to be helpful with something, what sort of help would that be?

MRS. DUQUESNAY: [Touching her husband's shoulder gently] Well, since they are saying that nothing shows up—I mean, nothing shows up on the EEG—they don't think these are real seizures. We want whatever it would take to get him better. That is all I know. He doesn't like it, and I don't like it.

JLG: Is your understanding of what you are being told here today different from what you were told before you came here?

MR. DUQUESNAY: Well, I was treated for . . .

MR. DUQUESNAY: [Indignant] Seizures for 2 years, ever since 1988. Why this change all of a sudden? Why is it that all this time they have been treating him for seizures? Why did they say they were seizures, yet now they say they aren't seizures? It's hard to understand that. Do you know what I'm saying?

JLG: Exactly what were you told by your doctors here?

PIERRE: [The son] "Episodes."

MRS. DUQUESNAY: No, "spells."

MR. DUQUESNAY: "Spells." [Agreeing]

As I listened, I sought to keep my own inner dialogue within the bounds of the conversational domain, a language of "spells" and "bad nerves," not "pseudoseizures" and "anxiety disorder" drawn from the usual professional discourse about such problems. I was also mindful of my assumptions about the Duquesnay family and their problem—choosing to believe that Mr. Duquesnay genuinely wished to be free of his symptoms, that resolution of the problem was in fact possible, that he and his family held wisdom about the problem that needed to be heard and understood, that he and his family already possessed resources needed to solve the problem if they could learn how to access and use them. These assumptions were nonobligatory choices, made deliberately. It could have been as plausibly argued that the patient had no motivation to change, because he received too much positive reinforcement from his wife's efforts to comfort and soothe him or from the disability payments he was receiving for his seizure disorder; or that the family was so dysfunctional that it required his illness and disability in order to preserve its homeostasis; or that the family was too impoverished in its intellectual, educational, cultural, and financial resources to be able to use modern psychotherapy. Each of these alternative professional narratives about the problem could be forcibly argued, although no one of them, including my choice, could have been either proven or disproven by the evidence at hand. The important question was not which assumptions were in some sense most true, but which assumptions would so shape my own perceptual and cognitive processes, as a clinician, so that the growth of a therapeutic relationship would be most furthered.

JLG: You feel that the doctors here have not fully understood?
MRS. DUQUESNAY: [Angrily] They treat you like you don't know what you are talking about. They told him, "You should be able to stop them. . . ."
PIERRE: Like mind over matter. . . .
MRS. DUQUESNAY: But anybody who has watched him have a seizure . . .
MR. DUQUESNAY: Every time Dr. Day comes in, he upsets me. He says, "There is nothing wrong with you. It's all in your head."
MRS. DUQUESNAY: Jimmy can't stand for anybody to say he is faking, or he is lazy and doesn't want to work.
JLG: So right now, you feel you are in a position of disagreement with the doctors, the neurologists, here?
MRS. DUQUESNAY: I don't guess it is really a case of disagreement, Dr. Griffith. Some of this may be from depression and all that. But what I don't understand is, when he went into the hospital, he didn't go in for seizures! He went in for blackout spells and bad headaches. He had his first grand mal seizure after he went into the hospital. He didn't get the depression until *after* he got so sick, because Jimmy is an outdoor person, and he can't stand being shut up in the house. He is a worker. He can't stand a lazy person. Never has, has he, son? My kids will tell you that. That is just . . . I don't understand why a man . . .

In inquiring about conflict between Mr. Duquesnay and his neurologists, I pointedly did not inquire about "who is right" or "what is correct," but about differences in "positions." Mrs. Duquesnay responded in turn with complementary language, "a case of . . . ," rather than another blaming statement. The use of language to separate the person from the position sidesteps the triggering of alarm when conflict is discussed. These are examples of linguistic practices that expand, rather than constrict, the variety of problem-solving strategies than can be used.

JLG: It seems to me that even if you could get them to understand the heart of what you want them to understand, there would still be a problem to deal with.

MRS. DUQUESNAY: They don't understand . . .

JLG: But what if they did understand? What would you then be asking them in terms of what you want to accomplish here?

MRS. DUQUESNAY: Find out what is causing . . .

MRS. DUQUESNAY: Find out what is causing the seizures, and help me with them.

JLG: Okay.

MRS. DUQUESNAY: Well, really Dr. Griffith, he went through 6 months here, before he went into the hospital, when he might have had just two or three seizures during that time. He was doing well. The medicine was all right. He was doing better. He felt better. And he got sick . . . he got the flu, and I mean, it was sick, sick . . . he stayed in the bed about 3 weeks.

JLG: So you went 6 months almost having none?

MR. DUQUESNAY: Yeah.

JLG: So this is not the way you usually are?

A patient's story as told by a biomedical inquiry invariably casts the illness as the protagonist with the patient a supporting actor. It is important to ask questions that reverse the figure and ground, setting the healthy patient as protagonist and his everyday life-style as the landscape, into which the illness temporarily intrudes. The 6 months of no seizures is transformed into his usual manner of living, rather than is his recent decompensation.

MRS. DUQUESNAY: During that time he got better, a lot better. The kids talked about how much better he was.

JLG: So you don't have any idea how things got bad again?

MRS. DUQUESNAY: When he got sick. They said he had the flu, and he stayed really sick for days and days. He stayed in the house. He didn't get out. He didn't want to see anyone.

MR. DUQUESNAY: I didn't want to talk to anybody.

MRS. DUQUESNAY: And something else that his doctors did not notice. They had changed his nerve medicine two or three times during that period of time, because he was shaking really badly and his nerves were too bad.

JLG: Have the medication changes had an effect on things?

MR. DUQUESNAY: I don't know.

MRS. DUQUESNAY: It has an effect on him. He is really irritable now.

MR. DUQUESNAY: I've tried to tell these doctors.

MRS. DUQUESNAY: But they were so concerned with these seizures that they . . .

MR. DUQUESNAY: [Gesturing vigorously] As I told Dr. Winston, "I also have headaches!" And he said to me, "So? Even I have headaches."

MRS. DUQUESNAY: But Jimmy is a man with cluster headaches. That is different, isn't it?

PIERRE: [Leaning forward, gesturing forcefully with his arm] Not everybody, like Daddy, has headaches constantly, all the time!

MRS. DUQUESNAY: Not to where they put him out . . . he can't stand sounds . . . a dark room is all he wants, with a rag on his head. . . . I mean, he can't cope. Because they really put him out, as long as he has the headache. But when he doesn't have the headaches—and they do let up sometimes—he is all right. He goes visiting. He gets out of the house. He loves to walk.

[Mr. Duquesnay, listening, reaches to hold his head.]

JLG: [Looking puzzled] So were you largely free of headaches during this 6 months you weren't having seizures?

MRS. DUQUESNAY: Yeah.

MR. DUQUESNAY: Pretty close!

JLG: So were you wishing they would focus more on the headaches and less on the seizures?

MR. DUQUESNAY: Well, it seems to me that the headaches could be a lot of my problem, and the doctors are not checking them out.

JLG: So if you had better control of the headaches . . . ?

MRS. DUQUESNAY: That doctor said to the nurses this morning when she came in there, "You all are still giving him the Vistaril [a mild, nonaddicting drug for anxiety] for his head, aren't you?" But the Vistaril doesn't seem to be making any difference. Especially when he has a seizure, he really has a headache after he wakes up.

MR. DUQUESNAY: The head neurologist, when he came in that day, he looked at me. He said, "Seems like we are not helping you. So what do you want us to do?"

MRS. DUQUESNAY: That is the part I don't understand. The treatment was helping him for that 6 months, up until he got sick. I don't understand it, really.

JLG: Did something change in how they were helping you?

MR. DUQUESNAY: The seizures? While down there at the neurology clinic?

MRS. DUQUESNAY: They increased his medicine.

MR. DUQUESNAY: They increased my medicine to get the blood levels up.

MRS. DUQUESNAY: A lot of Jimmy's problem is worry, because his medicine costs so much, and we don't have any insurance to help with it.

JLG: When you look at all these things you mentioned, which ones have you picked out that might be most related to things getting worse?

With each new shift, the story has become more complex. Now it is a story not simply of a man with pseudoseizures but of a man living with well-controlled seizures until poorly controlled headaches, multiple changes in medications, and worry over the cost of the new medications somehow interacted to create instability. Without their telling, I could never have guessed the specific interpretations and language with which they understood their situation—that Mr. Duquesnay experienced his doctors as viewing his failure to respond as "laziness" or that Mrs. Duquesnay's theory about his deterioration was that he was "an outdoor person" who had been involuntarily confined indoors by illness. These addenda to the narrative as originally told appear as the conversational participants drop their emotional postures of mobilization for those of tranquility.

Emotional postures of mobilization have as their drawback a narrowing of attention. Anyone who has looked for lost car keys when already late for an appointment, or tried in the dark to find the right key to fit a lock, is familiar with this kind of "tunnel-vision" that arises so easily to hinder effective problem solving when one is frustrated or afraid.

Emotional postures of mobilization select exclusionary language for their expression ("What is really going on is . . . "; "This is nothing more than . . . "; "All I know is . . . "; "It is either . . . , or . . . "). In their medical treatment, both the Duquesnay family members and their physicians had been recruited into "either/or" language that made it increasingly unlikely that an escape could be found from this unsatisfactory discourse. As an antidote to this kind of thinking, a clinician can use inclusive, "both/and" language, so that screened-out ideas and ignored events can receive attention ("One possibility could be . . . "; "One description of the problem would be . . . "; "One idea that comes to mind about this is . . . "; "Could it be both . . . and . . . ?") Here, detailed questioning from a "both/and" perspectives revealed a smorgasbord of possible events and situations that could plausibly be related to Mr. Duquesnay's worsening seizures.

MRS. DUQUESNAY: To be honest with you, I think it is a number of things, not just one thing. There were a bunch of things piled up together at one time.

JLG: Which were the most important ones that you think piled up together?

MRS. DUQUESNAY: I guess the worst one for him would be his headaches.

[Mr. Duquesnay nodded with his wife's words. As the son leaned forward, listening intently, I also leaned forward, mirroring his posture and speaking tentatively.]

JLG: The headaches got worse? Okay. What else?

MRS. DUQUESNAY: And his nerves are bad. And he has a lot of depression. Because Jimmy has never been the type to cry. Never, since we've been married. And lately, he gets upset easily. After the doctors had talked to him about his seizures, he didn't eat any supper last night or the night before that.

MR. DUQUESNAY: Yeah.

By this point in the interview, a patterning of family communication was visible: Whenever Mr. Duquesnay heard himself discussed in the third person, he adopted a shamed, sheepish facial expression and looked depressed. Here, as Mrs. Duquesnay continued to speak, he again lowered his head, hunched his shoulders, and wiped his forehead. His face showed resignation. Looking squarely into his face, I shifted the conversation to include him.

JLG: So the headaches got worse? And your nerves got worse? Right? And you had a number of medication changes. What were some of the other things that you think may have gone into the whole batch of things that may have been contributed to your condition getting worse? Were there other kinds of things?

[Mr. Duquesnay sat up, straightened, and spoke with a stronger voice.]

MR. DUQUESNAY: Well, depression . . . I stay depressed. I want to do something. I really want to do something. But I can't cope with being disabled. So I go to pieces.

JLG: It is really frustrating to you not to be able to do something active?

MR. DUQUESNAY: It sure is.

MRS. DUQUESNAY: You see, he has never been a house person, until he started having the blackout spells and stuff. And he will still get out there and try to work, even after he would almost pass out. He just hates being housebound. . . . He gets upset because he says, "You treat me like a child." But I really don't treat him like a child. The only thing I do is I don't leave him by himself. Because I come back and he is on the floor. You know.

JLG: As I said in the beginning, Melissa has been watching and listening to our conversation. What if I check in with her to get her impressions? Then we can talk some more after that.

An effective way to foster creative reflection is to structure the physical arrangement of a conversation in a manner that invites listening within emotional postures of tranquility. Employing the reflecting position in therapy is especially useful for this purpose. The use of reflecting techniques will be presented in greater detail in chapter 9. Here, the use of a reflecting team consultation for fostering creative listening and reflection by family members is demonstrated.

At my invitation, Melissa entered the room, and she and I then had a spontaneous, open discussion in front of the family members about what each of us had witnessed thus far during the interview.

After a friendly eye exchange and an explanation that the two of us would be talking with each other and that they could listen, we did not make further eye contact with them or engage them in the conversation. Our conversation in front of them occurred much as it would have occurred had we been discussing the case elsewhere.

[Melissa arranged our chairs, leaned back, relaxed, and paused a few seconds before speaking.]

JLG: Well, I know that it is a long and complicated story, but I wondered as you were watching and listening, if you had thoughts and ideas about the whole situation?

MEG: [Speaking slowly and softly, with gentle gestures punctuating the phrasing of her words] The thing that came through most clearly to me was something that seemed even more threatening to the Duquesnay family than the seizures—the idea that Mr. Duquesnay would be thought of by his doctors as lazy or "putting on." I wonder what it is really like amidst all his physical problems, to try to ensure that they believe he is a hard worker, that he doesn't want things this way, and that he is honest. These seem to be the most important things to me. It seems that they could put up with just about any kind of medical treatment, so long as the talk among the clinicians would not smack of accusations of laziness or putting on, these things that he hates so much.

I am sure it would bother anyone to feel accused of laziness. But I also wondered whether there were any parts in the history of their family life together, or in Mr. Duquesnay's own life, that would make this particular accusation feel so destructive. That's something I wondered about.

I also wondered what Mr. Duquesnay's father, or mother, or grandfather, or grandmother, or any of those people he grew up with, or his God, would say to him now as he lives in the middle of all this? I wondered, to whom could he look with confidence that they do know that he is doing the best he can? That must be the hardest thing. What do you think?

[As Melissa began to speak, Mrs. Duquesnay and Pierre reached out to place a hand on each of Mr. Duquesnay's shoulders, comforting him. Mr. Duquesnay's hands trembled, as he nodded agreement with Melissa's words.]

JLG: [Speaking more matter of factly, as in delivering a report] Well, I noted in particular that he talked about how hard it was not to have anything to do that was useful or productive when he stays in the house. It seems as if there are two levels of problems: First, what are these seizures and what can be done about them? It sounds like it has been quite oppressive to have them. But since he came into the hospital, a whole second set of problems arose, because of the way things have worked out in the doctor-patient relationships, where they have felt so misunderstood. It does not seem to me that they feel like they are on the same team that their doctors are on.

[Both Mr. and Mrs. Duquesnay leaned back, both appearing relaxed and lost in thought.]

MEG: Yes.

JLG: It must be like having two different problems to deal with. I am guessing that the second one—getting things worked out in their relationship with the doctors—has to be done before work really can begin on the other one.

[Mr. Duquesnay's hands began to tremble as he stared blankly into space, detached, appearing to drift into a trance. His wife and son gently shook each of his shoulders and called his name.]

MRS. DUQUESNAY: Jimmy! Jimmy! Hey!

[After a few seconds, Mr. Duquesnay looked around, made eye contact with his wife and son, and sighed deeply without speaking.]

MRS. DUQUESNAY: [To her husband] It will be all right!

MEG: [To JLG] Were there other thoughts you had as you listened and wondered?

[The three family members, recovering from the disruption, again turned to listen attentively.]

JLG: Only that I was struck by how puzzled they each seemed to be about this whole affair—that Mr. Duquesnay seemed to be healthy and strong and working and doing everything he wanted to do, then he started having the blackouts, and all this trouble began. Nobody seems to have a good explanation. Now they are in the hospital and feel as if they are being blamed, "It is your fault you are having these spells."

[Mr. Duquesnay, with a furrowed brow and pained expression, began to tremble again as he listened. His wife listened and nodded.]

MEG: Yes. And it does seem clear that they all really hate it.

[Melissa stood, smiled, and nodded respectfully to the family members, as she left again for the observation room. I then turned to the family members for their response to the conversation, asking what, if anything, struck their interest about our conversation.]

MRS. DUQUESNAY: When she said something about our hating it—we do all hate it, because we remember the kind of person Jimmy was before he got sick. And, you know, it affects the family to go through this stuff!

MR. DUQUESNAY: [Shaking his head as he spoke, no longer trembling] I couldn't ask for any better family.

MRS. DUQUESNAY: I can honestly say we have been very supportive of him.

MR. DUQUESNAY: [Emphatically] I couldn't ask for a better family!

MRS. DUQUESNAY: I'm not going to say that there haven't been some changes, because Pierre here was in the habit of going with his Daddy everywhere and doing things with him. He went through a hard time for about a year. He gave us fits, because he didn't know how to cope with his father being sick. They had quite a few rounds. But Jimmy showed him he was still Daddy, and he was still boss. And little by little Pierre realized. That doesn't mean he doesn't still have feelings about how things are, how Daddy can't do like he used to do.

But so far as coping is concerned . . . my daughters, they are unbelievable in how they are helping me. You don't know how many nights they have gotten up in the middle of the night and come into our bedroom to help me hold Jimmy on the bed, get him calmed down, and help change his clothes. All three of my kids have . . . the youngest is 14. . . . They love their Daddy. All of them do. My oldest girl is a "daddy baby" and always has been. She is her daddy's heart.

But the only time when he really does think we baby him is when I need to go somewhere to do things sometimes, or wish to, but I won't leave him at the house by himself.

[Pierre lowered his head, staring at the floor while his mother spoke.]

PIERRE: I guess we overprotect him sometimes, because we won't let him do anything alone, except go to the restroom and personal stuff like that. But, I mean, it is just like the other day when I was up here, me and him. He went to the restroom, and I stood outside. He slipped. I've always had a horror of that, my leaving him in there by himself and his falling. He can't help himself.

[As his son spoke, Mr. Duquesnay looked down, again appearing withdrawn and defeated.]

MRS. DUQUESNAY: I've learned that so many times. I would leave him alone at the house, and he would have a seizure while I was gone. That is the only reason we don't leave him by himself. It is not because we are trying to act like he's a baby . . . we just care. Right, Jimmy?

MR. DUQUESNAY: [Nodding] Right.

From the therapeutic perspective of structural family therapy, the wife's repeated speaking for the husband and the family's description of their anxious "seizure watching" would be manifestations of the enmeshment and overprotectiveness that characterize a "psychosomatic family." From a behavioral perspective, many of their descriptions would point to family behavior strongly reinforcing the patient's sick role. From a psychoanalytic perspective, the patient's secondary gains from his illness would constitute gratification of infantile yearnings for dependency. Insofar as each could fit the reality witnessed, any one of these descriptions would represent valid alternatives to our perspective. When we examine their epistemological structure, however, descriptions of family structure, contingencies of reinforcement, and psychodynamic formulations each prove to be professional narratives describing the patient and family from a viewpoint outside their experience of the problem. These professional narratives hide the patient's and family's authentic experience of dilemma from the clinician. Staying inside the family members' narratives, we see that the professional stories quickly become part of their dilemma. Now they feel that they must protect their husband and father against implicit stigma from the professionals' stories, while still seeking the professionals' aid for strange physical symptoms that they do not understand and are outside their control. Their story becomes one of isolation, stoic endurance, and sorrow.

> [Mr. Duquesnay, looking directly into my eyes, began gesturing forcefully and speaking firmly, showing more energy and animation than at any time during the session thus far.]

MR. DUQUESNAY: I always was a hard worker, even from my youth.

PIERRE: Always, always.

MR. DUQUESNAY: Not bragging or anything . . .

PIERRE: Sometimes if you watch him work . . .

MR. DUQUESNAY: [Gesturing emphatically] My Daddy was a worker. He's been dead 15 years. He was a working man.

MRS. DUQUESNAY: To be honest with you, Dr. Griffith, I think that something is causing his seizures, I really do. I've seen him have too many. I've sat and cried—he's sat and cried.

> He's the kind of person who won't let you tickle his feet . . . try to tickle his feet, and he'll knock you off the bed. He can't stand for you to touch his feet. But when he has these seizures, you can do anything you want . . . you can tickle both feet at the same time, and he would never know it. Really! It baffles me.

> I don't understand how the doctors say that they are not real. Jimmy's brother, John, is an EMT, and he has always been a rough type of guy, you know what I'm saying? He worked on ambulances for years. He can tell when people are putting on and when they ain't. John will tell you—he has been around Jimmy enough to know—he says these seizures are definitely real. John told me, "Don't let anybody kid you. I don't know what is causing them, but I know they are real."

> It makes you wonder whether the neurologists are just looking at the really big things, like the EEG and the MRI scans that didn't show anything. It makes me wonder sometimes if it isn't some little-bitty something—and they are so busy looking for the big things, they forget to really look for the little things. I don't understand it. I really don't understand it.

> [As his wife spoke, Mr. Duquesnay again lowered his head, becoming still, showing the same stance of defeat seen before. Then his posture straightened and his animation returned.]

MRS. DUQUESNAY: [Looking up, speaking firmly, with confidence] I believe some of it now, although not at the beginning . . . like the striking out during my sleep and the bad nerves ... some of it is probably psychological.

MRS. DUQUESNAY: I believe that too. Especially since the doctors explained to me what to look for. You can tell the difference when it is really a seizure and when it is like he is trying "to get back at" something. You know what I am saying? Like the hitting out ... I don't know ... that must mean that there is a lot of anger built up inside him.

JLG: How do you estimate it? Which part is which, do you think? I mean, if you take a stab at estimating which percent is psychological and which percent is neurological, what do you say?

MR. DUQUESNAY: [Nodding, speaking thoughtfully, making eye contact] I don't know. I think, I believe, a good portion of it is psychological ...

MRS. DUQUESNAY: [Interrupting] Right now ... Right now.

MR. DUQUESNAY: But it wasn't.

JLG: Not in the beginning?

MRS. DUQUESNAY: No.

MR. DUQUESNAY: Now.

JLG: But now depression, and frustration, and stuff like that make it worse?

MR. DUQUESNAY: It makes it worse. It didn't start it. I don't believe it is the actual cause.

JLG: So you believe you have two kinds of seizures, or two kinds of ...

MR. DUQUESNAY: [Interrupting] Problems.

JLG: Problems.

MR. DUQUESNAY: I believe that.

Mr. Duquesnay then talked about the problem that weighed heaviest on his mind—a planned move by the family to Natchez in order for Mrs. Duquesnay to be near her father who recently had been diagnosed with terminal cancer. Mr. Duquesnay disclosed to his family for the first time just how hard this move to Natchez would be for him. When 10 years old, he had been badly beaten up in a fight by a larger, much older boy. In anger, Mr. Duquesnay's father assaulted and nearly killed the older boy's father. For over a year, the Duquesnay family waited tensely to learn whether their father would be sent to prison for this attack in retribution. Although he was not imprisoned, the incident thereafter hung like a black cloud over Mr. Duquesnay, who felt stigmatized at his school. As soon as he turned 18, he left Natchez and swore an oath that he would never return to the city that disgraced his family. He had never broken this oath; but now he felt duty bound, as a husband, to support his wife by moving with her to Natchez.

JLG: [To the family members] Did you realize he had such bad memories of Natchez?

MRS. DUQUESNAY: I didn't realize how bad it was until here in the hospital. I always knew he would never go back there to live.

MR. DUQUESNAY: Things were bottled up inside me—things I didn't want to talk about or bring out.

MRS. DUQUESNAY: He's never been one to talk a lot. The only one he would really talk to was my brother, while my brother was alive.

JLG: Has there ever been anyone who really knew how strong your feelings were about Natchez?

MR. DUQUESNAY: Not until recently.

JLG: This is a tough spot for you as a family ... [to Mrs. Duquesnay] you know that your father is dying, and you want to be with him, but [to Mr. Duquesnay] you know it is so hard to go there that it may make you sick if you do go there to live.

MRS. DUQUESNAY: The children don't want to go there either. They like their schools here. So I talked it over with him before we decided to go. I thought he was fine with it 100% ... until now ... I thought he was. But inside myself I still feel obligated—you only have one mother and one father.

JLG: Have you all talked as a family about this being a really difficult dilemma and how best to work it out? How as a family do you talk together when you have a decision about something that has to be made, even though neither choice is a good one?

The two parents talked with each other about the pros and cons of moving. Again, it was clear that there was no good solution, yet a decision must be made. The family members all agreed to meet again to work out a solution.

After this interview, Mr. Duquesnay's nonepileptic seizures ceased, and he was shortly thereafter discharged from the hospital. Over the next week, with two more family meetings, the family decided together that they would move to Natchez. They did so, however, with full awareness that this would constitute an enormous emotional stress for their husband and father.

When Speaking Heals the Body

All clinicians have a small bundle of cases with stories similar to the story of Mr. Duquesnay. A patient is in dire straits from symptoms that are out of control, the usual medical and psychiatric treatments have failed to make any headway, a clinician conducts a single therapy session with the family, and the symptoms evaporate.

Despite these seemingly miraculous outcomes, each of us has hesitated (with a few exceptions) to publish these case descriptions, because it is so easy for the telling of the story to suggest conclusions that we believe are incorrect—that the curative power lay with the charisma of the therapist, that the specific intervention employed brilliantly "targeted" the symptom, that no other approach to solving the problem could have worked.

We have analyzed these cases, and they have shown consistent features that may give a clue as to why much could be accomplished quickly: Most were characterized by the occurrence of an extreme symptom that persisted despite intense and dogged efforts by those involved in the problem to change it. Common sense would have proposed that something different be tried, but those involved in the problem seemed unable to step out of unsuccessful, stereotyped ways of looking at, thinking about, and acting to resolve the problem. Symptom resolution occurred as ways were found in the interview—in structuring the setting, in the questions we asked, in the emotional postures maintained by the clinician—that enabled the interview participants to move from emotional postures of mobilization to emotional postures of tranquility, where creativity and openness to new ideas could occur.

It has seemed to be less the person of the therapist or what major intervention was employed (a question asked, a behavioral assignment to be completed, a therapeutic ritual to be enacted), or even which psychological theory was used to conceptualize the intervention, and more what happened so that a change in problem-solving behavior became possible when it had been obstructed until then. The story of Mr. Duquesnay is particularly edifying, because it is so apparent that there was no brilliant intervention, carefully crafted question, or behavioral homework to which the success of the session could be ascribed. Many of the questions asked were simple ones that conceivably could be asked within a variety of different theoretical frameworks for conducting psychotherapy: What do I need to know in order to understand the problem? What do you think needs to be done? Is what you are understanding from what you are being told here different from what you were told before you came here? If I were to have any useful input into the situation, what might that be? The conversation the two clinicians had in front of the family was spontaneous and unrehearsed, with no specific change in family behavior intended. Yet, the interview was remarkably successful, compared to those attempted by previously involved clinicians.

Although one might have a difficult time labeling specific actions of the clinician as significant interventions, it can be argued that this interview was a linguistically skilled encounter, different from any conversation that might have ensued had the Duquesnay family been talking with a friend, their pastor, their family physician, or many other mental health professionals from whom they might have sought help. The interview evolved out of numerous on-the-spot decisions made by the clinician during the session, based on detailed observations, using carefully selected language, and following an overarching theory about how symptoms change.

Although there were no efforts made to explain or to instruct, the questions asked did consistently create a place where the experience of the Duquesnay family—their descriptions, their stories, their explanations, their observations about their dilemma—could be fully articulated. Within some therapeutic perspectives, this work might be considered "joining with the family" or "establishing rapport." However, such perspectives hold an underlying assumption that neither of us shares—that a competent therapist should already have in place a blueprint for the solution that the patient or family need to implement; thus, "joining" or "rapport" is needed only to gain their cooperation and compliance so that the "real" therapy can begin with the clinician's intervention.

From the perspective presented here, creating a space for the patient's and family's story is not a preparation for the therapy, it is the heart of the therapy. A clinician in principle cannot possess a correct map for how the problem is to be solved, since such a map can only emerge out of the dialogue itself and is thus coauthored by all participants in the conversation.

By the end of the session obvious shifts in emotional postures among family members had occurred that moved away from the initial fear and protest toward trust and reliance. With these shifts, a therapeutic relationship evolved within which important life narratives were told for the first time—additional stories of pride in hard work, of a humiliating encounter with a cardiologist, of devotion by family members to a disabled father—that enabled understanding to occur. Among these life narratives was the story of an unspeakable dilemma in which Mr. Duquesnay, in deciding to move or not to move to Natchez, would either betray himself or betray his wife, but could speak neither with her nor with his children about the dilemma, lest he burden them. As his expression was unshackled, his seizures—for which he had nearly been removed from his home to permanent chronic psychiatric care—suddenly disappeared, even though the dilemma itself was as yet unchanged from before the session.

The clinician's choice to ask questions with the intention of disclosing a dilemma was significant for complex reasons, both for the clinician and for the family members. For the clinician, the inquiry-into-a-dilemma questions created an openness for the unexpected, while heightening respect for and minimizing pathologizing of the patient and family members. For the family members, these questions pointed to a place in their lives where choice was inevitable, even though none of the available choices was desirable. Awareness of the inevitability of change can be healing when patients and family members have blamed themselves for failing to stabilize an impossible situation. Through shared dialogue, without blame or self-reproach, facing the inevitable can be conducted together by family members with courage, grace, and compassion for one another.

This was judged to be successful, not by what insight the patient or family members gained, or what they learned, or even how they changed, but by the fact that the therapeutic conversation, once begun, was sustained until all was said that needed to be said, the family members expressing successfully their storied experience. It is the responsibility of the clinician to use language skillfully to enable this telling that could not have otherwise occurred.

CHAPTER 6

When Speaking One's Story Is Not Enough

WITH SOME MIND-BODY PROBLEMS, speaking the story of one's personal experience is not the needed solution. In these cases, the problem is not so much that a patient's personal expression has been silenced, but that a guiding narrative of the patient's life is intrinsically destructive in the binds it places on his or her body.

Alice, a 30-year-old woman with a problem of compulsive eating, had become pregnant at age 16. Her family, fearing she and they would be shamed in their local community, sent her secretly to live with distant relatives until the baby was delivered. Her present episodes of binging food were intimately tied to a deep sense of stigma ("I am a bad person, emblazoned with a scarlet letter I can never take off") that had evolved out of her experience of shame and exile. Although she was finally able to tell the story in therapy, the self-scorn and binging continued.

Mrs. King was a 50-year-old woman who sought treatment for bouts of laryngeal spasm during which she could speak only with a soft, raspy voice. She had noticed that the episodes occurred only during times of stress. A careful study of these "times of stress," however, showed that they specifically were moments when she sensed that others around her were doubting her competence. Connected to this sense of scrutinizing judgment were stories from her growing up as the only sister among brothers in a family with strong gender roles. Their family traditions valued the males' assertiveness and independence but devalued the females' interdependence and concern with relationships. Understanding this historical context of her symptoms intrigued her, but its articulation and her self-understanding did not resolve her symptoms.

Kay, an attractive and stylish 25-year-old woman suffering from severe bulimia, stated, "It doesn't matter what men say. What they want is thin, thin, thin." At times she could reflect on the story of her childhood, when she learned to fear obesity after years of listening to her mother and sisters and watching movies and television commercials. But her understanding and talking about these influences did little to weaken their grip on her life.

For Kay, Alice, and Mrs. King, speaking their story did not necessarily diminish its power. It was not the expression of their old story, but the creation of a new story that was needed. We can contrast their stories with the dilemma that bound Mr. Duquesnay. For him, speaking itself was an act of rebellion. As an ill patient, he felt lost on a medical battlefield, at the mercy of back-and-forth fighting between his illness and nurses, doctors, therapists, hospitals, insurance companies, and government agencies warring against it. Distanced from his own body and alienated from his personal experience, he had lost a sense of authorship for the drama within which he was living. Life had become a series of terrors that appeared without warning or explanation, like a bad dream. Then the simple act of claiming a voice in the discourse, by speaking the story of his experience of the problem and insisting it be heard and understood, was itself therapeutic. His personal narrative changed from "I have no voice" to "I have a voice, and it is heard and understood." This change in life-narrative had important biological consequences in how it coordinated the physiological states of his body. This was the needed change that enabled healing to occur.

When this silencing of personal discourse is not the heart of the problem so much as is the quality of the narrative, creating a context for expression may not, alone, be sufficient to resolve the problem. As clinicians, we all know situations in which telling, listening, and understanding are not enough, because the stories available to the patient or the family members are devoid of effective ideas for dealing with the problem, or because available stories are intrinsically destructive ones that blame or disempower the patient or others in a manner that engenders suffering.

Locating Self-Narratives That Ensnare and Bind

Self-narratives are those stories of personal experience that define one's sense of selfhood, "who I am as a person" (Gergen & Gergen, 1983). We typically can identify specific self-narratives that are intimately connected to a somatic symptom, because they hold the patient within a double bind that silences expression of the body. These self-narratives often lie in the background of a patient's experience, however, cut off from the public discourse in which he or she easily engages in conversation. If we are to involve these self-narratives in the process of treatment, we must undertake a deliberate search to identify them, then, together with the patient, plan a strategy that undercuts their power. This is a process of deconstructing and externalizing self-narratives.

Deconstruction, a term borrowed from recent continental philosophy, refers to a process of rendering visible the hidden, interpretive assumptions that give meaning to an idea (Kearney, 1984; White, 1992). Often, these interpretive assumptions have been invisible, because they have become cut off from their historical origins as a specific truth belonging to a specific time and situation. Now they are assumed to be such generalizable truisms that they are assumed automatically, unseen and unquestioned in conversation.

For example, when we deconstruct an idea, such as Kay's statement that, "It doesn't matter what men say. All they want is thin, thin, thin," we seek to display openly the bundle of personal and cultural narratives that give weight to these statements during Kay's daily life. We want to reestablish the limitations of the specific context within which the narratives were born. Because these narratives are literally felt within the body, we begin their deconstruction with Kay's experience of her body. We ask: Just before you notice the urge to binge on food, exactly what do you feel in your body? If you were to imagine your body as being poised or readied for some kind of action or expression in relation to people around you, what might that be? We thus identify the characteristic emotional posture that is wedded to her symptom and ask her to name it.

We then inquire about which self-narratives are bound to this emotional posture: What are the important parts of life experience tightly connected to this specific emotion? Typically, a patient has no difficulty in telling several critical narratives of life experiences whose emotion joins that of the present moment.

The process of deconstruction next moves outward to inquire how various cultural, political, and religious practices gave form to these critical life experiences: What ideas about men and women most guided how you interpreted this critical experience in your life? How were you taught that these were valid ideas? What were other ways in which these ideas instructed you to think about or act toward yourself? When you witness how these ideas and their practices influence the lives of other women, do you see them as freeing or as subjugating? For yourself and the women you love—your sisters, daughter, and women friends—would you prefer to be guided by these ideas, or would you prefer different ones? What other sources of knowledge about yourself as a woman have you located in your life? How did you discover these other sources of knowledge? How would they have led you to regard your body differently?

Concurrently, externalizing questions are asked that separate the self-narratives and their cultural practices from the patient's selfhood. Externalization was developed by Michael White and David Epston as a therapeutic process that counters the power of social practices to embody pathology within persons (White & Epston, 1990). Externalizing questions name the processes of perception, cognition, or action that maintain a problem and inquire about their effects on a person, thus separating cleanly a sense of the problem and a sense of self as a person. Further questions personify these processes, as if they were a powerful enemy with malevolent intent and a crafty, seductive, deceitful character, or else a well-intended but misguided, controlling life manager: Do you remember a time before these stories of "chubby Kay" came into your life? Did these stories of "chubby Kay" seem to cloud or shed light on who you really are as a person? [If "cloud"] Once these stories came to cloud your vision, which aspects of yourself as a person did it become difficult to see? Have you missed being able to experience these parts of yourself? Can you imagine by what intent these stories would seek to hide your talents and abilities from your eyes? Have there been any ways of living that you might consider to be regrettable "bad habits" that these stories have led you into?

If such a self-narrative can be externalized, then the sources of its power can be more easily deconstructed; the more the sources of power become deconstructed, the more external to the patient's sense of selfhood that power becomes. By naming and drawing them into focus, the patient's dilemma and the narratives sustaining it are objectified. Then, in the emotional distance created, openings can be sought through which the patient can escape his or her dilemma and the symptom it brings.

This is a reversal of the usual process that has been occurring, in which the patient has experienced the self as objectified by the dilemma and accompanying self-narratives ("I am a bulimic"). White and Epston based externalization on one of the favorite strategies of the deconstructionist philosophers—the turning of a cultural practice upon itself in order to disable it. As such, externalization is a process heavy with irony. Its thrust is to separate problems from persons and to pathologize problems, not patients. To do so, however, it must identify, name, and flesh out into as-if-persons, these manners of living that one would ordinarily speak about in impersonal terms. The patient villifies and strikes out against an externalized manner of living and thereby avoids attacking herself or himself or another person.

As this deconstructive inquiry proceeds, clear and succinct descriptions of dilemmas and forced choices begin to be articulated. The patient discovers that the self-narrative gave rise to dilemmas in which he or she was compelled to make a choice, where each possibility was unacceptable and where conversation about the dilemma was proscribed. "You say that if you did not lose weight, then your family and friends would notice nothing about you except the shape of your body. But the discipline of losing the weight forced you to learn to notice nothing about yourself except your weight, and you couldn't even talk about it with your parents and friends. Was that the dilemma for you?"

Finally, it is usually important to ask questions that sensitize a person to the significance of living within the constraints of an unspeakable dilemma. Like citizens living under a totalitarian political state, patients learn to adapt to their dilemmas. One way to adapt is to develop amnesia for what life was like before the dilemma came. Another is to habituate to the hardship, so that the experience of dilemma does not seem burdensome. Still another is to learn to focus only on immediate problems, "taking it one day at a time," so that accruing, long-term consequences of living within the dilemma are not noticed. For example: "If your skill in seeing nothing about yourself except your body shape were to become even more perfected, what else about yourself as a person might you start to learn to ignore? Before bulimia entered your life, who knew you well, and what might they notice about you now as a person that your vision presently is obscured from seeing? If you were to have a daughter 15 years from now who began to fall into these same practices of bulimia, what would be the tell-tale signs that she was losing awareness of how much it was controlling her life? If these stories of 'chubby Kay' continue to influence your life, what will they likely guide you to do next? Will this be a loss that you would notice or not?" The rich elaboration of clinical techniques for asking reflective questions that recently has characterized family therapy can be productively applied throughout the stages of this process (Andersen, 1991; Epston, 1992; Penn, 1985; Tomm, 1987a, 1987b; White, 1986).

In practice, the sequence of questioning we outline here does not follow a rigid order, although the order presented here possesses a logical coherence. Once the relevant stories that coordinate symptoms have been identified, questions that articulate, deconstruct, and externalize dilemmas and sensitize patients and families to the long-term consequences of their dilemmas are intermixed according to the flow of conversation. This process can be outlined as:

1.) Identifying the characteristic emotional posture that is associated with symptom occurrence through detailed questioning about the state of the body when the symptom reliably occurs or is likely to occur.

2.) Asking questions that retrieve dominant self-narratives that anchor this emotional posture.

3.) Asking questions that externalize these self-narratives and their dilemmas.

4.) Asking questions that heighten the awareness of these binds and forced choices in the patient's life.

5.) Asking questions that sensitize the patient to the long-term consequences of living within an unspeakable dilemma.

A Map for Therapy

In this therapy, the clinician's participation is that of a consultant helping the patient and family members to study how the dilemma and its sustaining narratives operate. They learn to track the habits of the dilemma much as a farm family would study the habits of a fox raiding their chicken coop. When the dilemma and its stories are well understood, there usually appear quite obvious courses of action that can undercut their power. Often, there are a multitude of effective actions that can be taken, for if the mind-body problem is born of a rigidly unspeakable dilemma, there will be many different aspects of the situation that, if altered, will unravel either the silencing or the dilemma itself.

Although each binding story is unique, we can distinguish four paths that, separately or intertwined, seem to fit most of the ways in which patients and families escape these binds in our clinical work:

1.) The patient learns to stay away from situations that feed the power of a binding story. The patient and family members learn which circumstances and relationships to avoid because they are too risky.
2.) The patient locates a story from his or her life experience that evokes an emotional posture that blocks the occurrence of the symptom.
3.) The patient locates a nonbinding story that can displace the current binding story, either accessing an alternative story that has been lying fallow outside awareness or creating a new one.
4.) The patient reauthors an old binding story into a new form that does not create an unspeakable dilemma.

An overall map of therapy is described schematically in figure 6.1. Chapters 3 through 5 described steps for creating a conversational domain in which an unspeakable dilemma and the narratives surrounding it can be articulated safely. This chapter and chapters 7 and 8 describe ways for helping a patient and his or her family escape self-narratives that sustain a symptom even after the dilemma has been publicly expressed.

Deliverance from a Haunted Body

Escaping the influence of a story does not mean telling a patient that the story is false or that it makes no sense or that we have a different story that is more valid. We know that a "story" as many people think of it—written sentences in the pages of a book—is only an artifact, a token that stands for the story as it lives biologically as a dance of social interactions among the members of a

Figure 6.1
A MAP FOR THERAPY

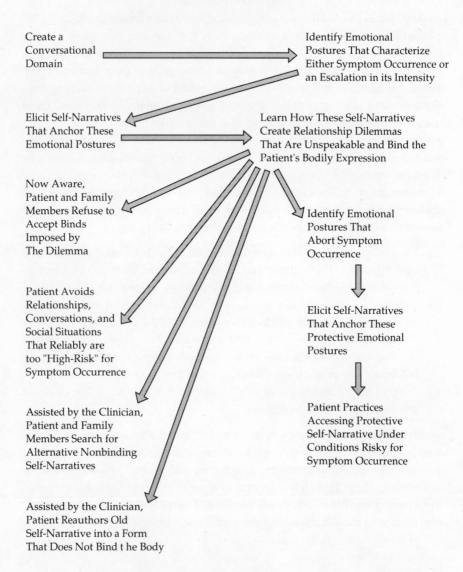

family, clan, or society. We also know that stories are supported by social practices—the customs, politics, rituals, and other habitual ways that shape how people live together. Escaping the influence of a story means that we must challenge it where it exists in the patient's lived experience, in the habits and social practices of daily life that embody it.

Our task is a search for counterpractices, effective antidotes that disable a destructive story's bind on the body. These are new habits, rituals, and life-styles that obstruct participation in a destructive story. Frances, dying from bulimia, defied her family lore ("Whatever you must do, don't tell Mama because it would kill her") to compose a letter to her mother about the childhood abuse Frances had suffered. Ms. Martin, suffering from intractable headaches, developed a habit of systematic inquiry as to what her body was experiencing—What am I feeling? Where do I feel it in my body? How do I name this emotion? I am experiencing this emotion in regard to whom? Mrs. Jackson, also suffering from headaches, challenged her childhood learning that "it is better to keep your mouth shut" by consistently speaking with her husband about her inner dilemmas as they appeared in her daily life.

The design of a counterpractice might seem to be a task for the therapist, because a good therapist must know how to prescribe behavioral assignments that accurately target specific problems. Much clinical work among strategic therapists, hypnotists, cognitive-behavioral therapists, and solution-focused therapists does rely on the creativity of the therapist for designing clever and elegant assignments that, when executed, undercut a symptom. In our work, however, we have been repeatedly surprised and delighted by the creativity with which patients and their families located their own specific counterpractices among life skills already possessed. Just as research pharmacologists scour the earth looking for new antibiotics among enzymes that fungi, molds, and other plants already produce, instead of trying to compose new molecules de novo in the laboratory, we go on similar wide-ranging searches with persons looking for previously unnoticed skills that stand ready to counter a binding self-narrative.

A good place to begin is an inquiry about where, when, and how a destructive self-narrative shows itself in a person's life. Which conversations, relationships, and life situations tend to resurrect it? Are there situations where its apparent power is so great that the person, at least for the present, should avoid them? What are the best arguments the self-narrative can offer to convince the person of its validity? If there are moments of weakness when the person feels most vulnerable to the influence of the self-narrative, how are these moments best characterized? These questions are a study in the anthropology of a narrative: They stalk the self-narrative to learn its ways within the person's life-world.

These questions also assign the self-narrative a name and personify it with human qualities. Personifying a self-narrative as an adversary brings an immediate shift in the emotional postures of the body, from those of entrapment—either fearful protest or apathetic detachment—to those of rebellion—defiance, assertion, outrage. For example, Victor was a middle-aged man who was awakened in the middle of the night by a sense of being strangled, terrifying chest pains, and shortness of breath that he thought to be a heart attack, until an evaluation in a sleep disorders laboratory showed them to be nocturnal panic attacks. He would lie paralyzed in fear each night until the pain passed.

The mystery and the tactics of the pain were exposed when he connected these bodily feelings with the threats of an older man who forcibly molested him at a carnival one night during his childhood. As Victor told of this act, he remembered the man's threat. I (MEG) recorded the exact words he attributed to the fear, to the man, and the words about light he used for himself and his strength.

In externalizing and personifying the fear, I recalled Victor's words: "The fear that startles you in the middle of the night . . . that tries to strangle and paralyze you . . . that reminds you of the awful pain that says you are small and weak and to be used . . . that says, 'If you ever tell, I will kill you' . . . how does this fear stand up to the light? Does it shrink into the shadows, waiting for you to forget your strength, to forget that you have spoken now, to forget what you know now that tells you that you are not alone? What will you keep with you through the night that will remind you that the light is within you, always with you?" This shift, from experiencing fear as a vague, inanimate, abstract entity to a hostile, attacking, humanlike creature, enabled the reconfiguration of Victor's attentional and information-processing systems and his muscles, glands, and cardiovascular system to be readied for aggression, instead of passive submission. Victor's chest pains ceased when he found language to externalize and to personify his fear.

Such an emotional reposturing of the body happens as soon as the language changes, even before the patient takes concrete actions based on the new perceptions. In a significant number of other cases, too, this change in body state alone has been sufficient to disengage the somatic symptom, even before a treatment plan for altering behavioral patterns could be implemented.

Two Different Notions of "Story"

In talking about self-narratives as entities that we can split away from a person's life, we are alternating between dual definitions of "story." The distinction between the two is important. Until now, we have spoken about a story, including a self-narrative, as a linguistic unit of coordinated bodily states among members of a social group. In this biological sense, stories exist within the dance of bodily interactions among the group members. But in speaking about a self-narrative as an objectlike entity to be named, externalized, and deconstructed, we speak about the self-narrative as created out of the living dance of bodily interactions.

To name a story is to step out of it. A named story is an artifact. Like the skin of a snake that we find in the grass, long after the living snake has slithered away, a self-narrative cannot be named, objectified, and manipulated and still be experienced as the vibrant, flowing story within which the person lives. What we have done is more analagous to making a videotape of a day in a person's life that we can then cut and splice until, in our editing together, we have created a coherent story of the life. The person's life has, of course, moved on according to its own direction, oblivious to our efforts to catch a piece of it on film. Yet, the impoverished product of our art may be extraordinarily helpful if that person, inspired by our film, undertakes a reflective retelling of his or her life story that is richer in its possibilities than the self-narrative previously lived within.

It is important to us that we can employ this process to create turbulence in the flow of a destructive self-narrative as it is lived out in the moments of a patient's daily life. Each of us experiences ourselves limited in scope of power and personal agency, at least to some extent, whenever we are labeled as male or female, white or black, American or Asian, young or old. We can turn this process of objectification on binding self-narratives by creating from them visible pieces of art that, beheld by the patient, inspire him or her to create new ways of living that incapacitate the binding self-narrative.

In broad strokes, we can describe the clinical approach in the chapters 4 and 5 as hands-on therapeutic work with binding self-narratives as they exist in the moment-to-moment movements of the patient's life. In working directly with this living story of a person's life, we can do no more than ask questions and create therapeutic contexts that invite creative change. Such change cannot be prescribed, directed, or predicted.

The present work, on the other hand, is better described as ways to create storied artifacts out of a patient's lived experience that can be reworked in ways that subsequently open new possibilities for healing. We can handle these lifelike artifacts in ways we plan to be therapeutic, much as an artist may carefully select color, line, and shape to create a painting of a city that purposefully invites an emotion of contentment, anger, or anomie in the viewer.

Challenging Assumptions That Have Silenced Alternative Self-Narratives

Building a new life-style based on resisting an externalized self-narrative enacts a new, alternative life story. Patients who have lived much of their lives with destructive self-narratives and the problems they promulgated often have lost sight of their ability to identify, to interrogate, and to challenge the authority of the stories that guide their lives. When we first met him, Mr. Duquesnay, for example, had no sense that he had a choice as to which stories he would live within. As with Mr. Duquesnay, one uniform aspect of such new stories has been a theme of freedom from secrecy:

Although one may be trapped by circumstances, one will not be trapped in silence. The dilemma can be expressed in language, rather than in the body's performance.

One can help deconstruct a patient's assumptions about reality that function to silence his or her personal expression. In creating a conversational domain, optimal conditions have already been set for the telling of personal stories. Actions by the therapist to structure a setting and to create the kind of conversation and relationship that facilitate emotional postures of tranquility may be sufficient for self-narratives of significance to be expressed. But when this telling remains difficult or impossible, it may be necessary to articulate, externalize, and deconstruct any beliefs, interpretations, or assumptions that hinder the expression of experience.

For example, Keith, a young addictionologist, wondered if he had chronic fatigue syndrome, because he always felt so chronically tired and tense. He felt baffled and disappointed, because his symptoms appeared soon after he gained the job he had longed for, and, despite his fatigue, medical testing could provide no answer. He feared that his lethargy would have a detrimental impact on his young son. Keith's mother, a severe alcoholic, had died the year before. Although some in the family were relieved by her death, Keith missed her.

When I (MEG) asked about times Keith and his mother spent together, Keith would preface his stories with, "I know I was codependent with my mother, but. . . " It seemed that all of his caring and loving memories of his mother were filed away under "codependency" or, if they were very happy memories, under "denial." Who would be categorizing their relationship in this way, I wondered? Had Keith responded that only his siblings or only his colleagues had seen things this way, it would have been simpler to deconstruct. But Keith himself also made this judgment. He was concerned that enjoying some of the memories of his mother might tumble him back into the dark hole of codependency. Yet he wanted to honor his mother and to keep her in his heart.

The 12-step recovery language of "denial" and "codependency" had been lifesaving for Keith in his own alcoholism, and he now employed it to help others. He did not want to depart from his understanding of the alcoholic family system. But within its language, he could find no way to hold the memory of his mother dear. He either could keep his recovery intact or keep the memories of his mother intact, but not both.

I asked what Keith's mother had been like before she was an alcoholic. Which parts of his mother's character, personality, and behavior had remained resilient to the effects of the alcoholism? Were there times in between the drunken times when the mother he loved showed through?

"If we weren't talking . . . if you were just quiet, remembering the happy times with your mother through your senses . . . does your nose know what you would smell, do your eyes know what they would see, do your ears know what they would hear?"

Keith was quiet, breathing slowly as he sat. "My mother used to make us this wonderful stew. The ingredients would surprise you. You wouldn't think it would be good, but it was. As I asked him the recipe, he added, "I can almost smell it now."

"Would you like to taste it again?" I asked.

"Yes. I think I'll make some for my wife and son. I'll do it Saturday."

"As you are in the kitchen stirring the stew, enjoying the smell, how would you like to imagine your mother?" I asked.

"I want to think of Mama cooking and laughing and being happy to serve us that good stuff, because that's how she was then."

Keith made the stew the next Saturday with his son, and decided to serve it at every Christmas dinner. He then found other ways to enjoy memories of his mother, such as the music they both had loved. He became comfortable talking about this nonalcohol-centered relationship he shared with his mother.

Keith's energy and zest for living began to return, and his complaints of fatigue faded. In his work, he found he had a more complex appreciation of his alcoholic patients than did many of his colleagues because of his ability both to confront them about their addiction and to enjoy them as persons.

When Keith first appeared for therapy, "alcoholic" and "codependent" had become ideas so closely held that they were no longer ideas but an all-inclusive worldview. They offered to Keith all there was to be known about his mother, himself, and their relationship. Through indirect questioning that elicited aspects of his mother and their relationship unsullied by alcohol, the clinician by implication relegated "alcoholic" and "codependent" back to a status as one set of interpretive ideas among others. As a desirable, but unanticipated consequence, Keith also began to appreciate his ability to perceive aspects of his patients that lay outside their identities as "alcoholics."

Geographic Escapes from Binding Stories

Sometimes the solution to a mind-body problem lies in staying away from life situations that reliably resurrect powerful stories that sustain the symptom. During the era of psychoanalytic therapies, it was axiomatic that the central objective for therapy should be the kind of character change that ideally renders one invulnerable to the vicissitudes of life circumstances. For example, a "well-analyzed" person supposedly could go to a family reunion full of unresolved, conflictual, grief-filled relationships without experiencing the sudden pain of a headache or the spasm of a duodenal ulcer. Such an emphasis on character change, rather than symptom relief, labels the simple avoidance of circumstances that trigger symptoms as complicity with one's psychopathology. Posing character change as the standard solution, however, fails to recognize that many life dilemmas arise out of injustices and threats of harm, not a deficit of character. Revising character in this manner may also be far too time-consuming and expensive than a patient's resources permit and is generally not what the patient is requesting. As our objective is symptom relief, competent life management may include prudent choices not to expose oneself to situations where the configuration of relationships or cultural politics prescribe unspeakable dilemmas.

For example, Robert Johnson was a 56-year-old man who was hospitalized because of weakness and numbness that occurred suddenly over the right side of his body. In the hospital, he told me (JLG) the story of the relationship with his older brother, Samuel, who, unasked by Robert, had assumed an authoritative and paternal role toward his younger brother after their father, years earlier, had died. Samuel had an explosive temper that since childhood had led to outbursts of cursing and fighting with family, friends, coworkers, and acquaintances. When younger, Robert had felt physically intimidated by Samuel's aggressiveness. Now Samuel was ill and weak in his old age. Still, however, he verbally castigated and humiliated Robert whenever they differed. Robert found that he no longer could bear the resentment and humiliation of the countless stories that boiled within him when assailed by Samuel. He was afraid that he would lose control of his own temper and seriously injure his older brother if they were to come to blows, and he knew that he could not control for long his rage when verbally assaulted by Samuel. Robert also realized that he could never talk about this issue openly with Samuel, because Samuel's reaction to the perceived criticism would be so vitriolic that the discussion probably would trigger the very fight that Robert most wanted to avoid. In the midst of this dilemma, Robert's right arm and leg became weak and numb.

In the hospital, I gathered Robert's immediate family members and a trusted friend for a conference. As they talked about the dilemma that Robert faced with his older brother, the different persons offered a variety of suggestions about what could be done. In the end, Robert, his wife, and their adult daughter all agreed that the wisest course would be to move away from the family home where Samuel still lived. All Robert's family members and his close friend agreed that attempting conversation with Samuel about the issue was out of the question. If, for the sake of his health, Robert needed to exclude from his life these present and past stories of humiliation and domination by his brother, then he needed to stay away from him. After the decision to move was made, Robert's paralysis and numbness resolved within the day.

Just as a person struggling to overcome alcoholism may for a time avoid dining with friends who serve wine with dinner, so may a person struggling against a disabling self-narrative choose to stay away from, at least for a time, those relationships and situations that conjure up its presence. It is important to show appropriate respect for the power of a story, just as one would respect the power of any adversary, even while making plans to confront the adversary.

Finding Stories That Protect and Heal the Body

Choosing to examine destructive stories to learn how to avoid them carries an important implication, that a choice has also been made to live within a new, alternative story. For Mr. Duquesnay, this new story was one of having a voice that would be heard. For Robert Johnson, it was one of refusing to cower before his older brother. These preferred, alternative stories can be sought explicitly from the beginning. Such a search shifts our attention away from the domain of the problem to a domain of possible solutions. This shift marks a watershed in our clinical work, across which our clinical methods switch from defending against the influence of destructive stories to aggressively displacing destructive stories with better alternatives that promote healing. This is a shift from a problem focus to a solution focus.

A direct and powerful way to locate self-narratives that are in the truest sense protective and healing is to employ the same method used to locate the self-narrative associated with the symptom, but to follow it in the opposite direction. As one self-narrative can hold the body in a bind, so can another so position the body that a symptom is unable to appear.

The simplest way to locate healing self-narratives is to ask: "Is there a particular state of your body, a particular emotion, within which your symptom would *never* occur?" If this emotional posture can be described in detail and given a name, then one next asks: "What are the critical parts of your life story that are tightly connected to this emotion?" Usually, a person can quickly identify a number of powerful experiences that, in their telling, bring the body into a protective emotional posture.

John B. was a 46-year-old attorney who described episodes of debilitating esophageal spasms since his early teenage years. Now the spasms mainly occurred when competing demands from multiple projects at work made him frustrated and resentful. They caused excruciating cramping pains in his chest, which had been at first frightening but now were something to stoically endure. Although he found benefits in other areas of his life, several years of psychodynamic psychotherapy and additional training in progressive muscle relaxation had each failed to improve these symptoms. Some antispasmodic medications brought partial relief, but no medicine had completely relieved the spasms, except narcotics, which were unacceptable for long-term use.

In telling the story of his symptoms, John described how he had that week suffered through a siege of pain that began on a day when he was rushing between two projects, for neither of which he could produce his best work. I (JLG) questioned John carefully about the specific emotional posture out of which the spasms arose: Were there any signs he could notice among all the events and relationships around him that would tell him that this would be a time of risk for his spasms to begin? "Describe exactly what you notice in your body that signals to you that a spasm is building. As these sensations begin to build and build, what would your body say if it could be given a voice?" If he were to think of these sensations as a part of his body getting ready for some kind of action, what kind of action would that be? Where or toward whom would it be directed? What words would he use to name the emotion that fits these sensations?

This questioning identified "shame" as the dominant emotional posture out of which his symptoms arose. However, it was a shame with very specific characteristics, as a bodily state that arose when John felt himself judged, in his eyes or those of others, to be inadequate, to be one who has failed to provide enough for the commitments he had made.

I then asked John which parts of his life story were most tightly connected to this specific emotional posture. After only a brief pause, he told several stories from when he was 10 to 12, at which age, after the death of his father, he became the man of the house for his mother who was overworked and chronically ill. He then had often felt this same bodily sense of inadequacy and shame.

I next asked whether there might be an emotional posture in which his symptoms could never occur. Was there an emotional posture that would instead bring comfort to the sensations of inadequacy and shame? And what were the parts of his life story that connected most tightly with this emotional posture? John responded with two very different kinds of self-narratives, both of which brought a deep warmth and relaxation that he felt in his chest.

First, he talked about how it felt to be touched and held in lovemaking by a woman who he knew loved, accepted, and desired him. He particularly remembered the kisses, caresses, and conversations with a girl at age 14 who loved him, as he now looked back, with perfect innocence. Second, he remembered some moments when his mother lay dying when he knelt on the floor beside her bed, weeping and holding only her hand in his, caressing it with his lips and feeling the veins of her hand against his cheek.

John entered deeply into either of these two narratives by recollecting vividly the scene, the words spoken, the colors, the smells, the sensations of touch. He entered an emotional posture of "joyful acceptance," with bodily sensations of a warm fullness, a deep, visceral relaxation, and a focused awareness only on the presence of the beloved that he imagined. The first story was one of tender and passionate acceptance by a woman; the second a story of giving to a woman all that it was possible for devotion to give.

Despite the chronicity and past intransigence of his esophageal spasms, John henceforth found that he could reliably abort his spasms in their pro-dromal stages by entering into one of these self-narratives, or one of their associated vignettes, thereby gaining access to its emotional posture of joyful acceptance and the recoordination of bodily state that this emotional posture brought. He was able to discontinue most use of medications for the problem.

John's days were filled with business expectations from clients that were functional in nature. They were interested in what he could produce, whether it was delivered on time, and whether it was of good quality. This relationship world stood ready to validate his old self-narrative of inade-quacy and shame that he could not do more, do it faster, or do it better. However, a different but complementary self-narrative lay latent within him, about a man whose deepest joy was to give and to know acceptance in the eyes of the other. The first self-narrative coordinated a shrinking and tightening down of his body, as if under a judging gaze, readying his body to hide or disappear; the second self-narrative coordinated an opening and relaxing of his body to receive the touching and caressing of another who knew no judgment but only love. Both were possibilities for his mind and body at any given moment, depending on which story he chose to enter. More important, this possibility was available to him despite the circum-stances of his harried workday, which were often entirely outside his con-trol, simply by momentarily leaving his interpersonal world and its conver-sations and entering his intrapersonal world with its conversation.

Identifying self-narratives that are protective, healing, and soothing are critical when a person is trapped in a real-life dilemma from which there is no visible escape. For family, political, or economic reasons, people do some-times find themselves involved in dilemmas for which a choice to end the destructive relationship seems unimaginable. For example, a double-bind relationship with one's child or parent may trigger somatic symptoms, yet ending the relationship is not an option that can be considered. Or one may suffer from bigotry and prejudice in one's community that brings somatic symptoms, yet the means are absent for moving out of that community. Or a double-bind relationship with a boss at work may trigger somatic symp-toms, yet one may feel so financially dependent on the job that tolerating its symptoms seems to be a price worth paying. Arlie Hochschild (1983, p. 17) has pointed out how the buying and selling of emotional labor is in fact an integral part of modern capitalism: "A nineteenth-century child working in a brutalizing English wallpaper factory and a well-paid twentieth-century American flight attendant have something in common: in order to survive in their jobs, they must mentally detach themselves—the factory worker from his own body and physical labor, and the flight attendant from her own feelings and emotional labor." When there are compelling reasons why a person must remain in a double-bind relationship that is certain to bring symptoms, the person's recourse lies with denying the social interaction the power to prescribe self-narratives that shape his or her bodily state. Although a particular situation or relationship can seem to compel a particular telling of a person's life story, it is yet possible for the person to turn away from the interpersonal dialogue to his or her inner dialogue for a more preferred story.

The recommendation to John was kin to aspects of the acting method pioneered by Konstantin Stanislavsky almost a century ago (Moore, 1991). Stanislavsky taught actors how to use emotional memory to create spontaneous and realistic emotions, rather than grimacing, twitching, staring, or sulking according to some formula in an attempt to affect the audience in a particular way. With emotional memory, an actor instead imagines in vivid detail a specific real-life experience that in the past generated an intense emotion. As the scene is imagined, the emotion spontaneously expresses itself in the actor's feelings and body. Thus, the actor neither mimicks the expression of authentic emotion nor attempts to will the emotion into being. Rather, he or she uses the "as-if" capability of the imagination to resurrect a memory or create a fantasy of being mugged, of winning a championship, of freezing in the snow, of being seduced by a lover, whereupon the expressed emotions of terror, elation, numbness, or passion spontaneously flow more convincingly real than if the actor tried to form the emotion directly. Another example illustrates how an inward vision can foster a return to health.

Ms. Nichols was a middle-aged woman who had been disabled throughout her adult life by somatization disorder, a chronic and severe syndrome of multiple kinds of somatic symptoms that wax and wane over time. Her symptoms had in fact improved remarkably over the course of a therapy during which she discovered a variety of relationships between life stresses and occurrence of her symptoms and developed some appropriate strategies for protecting her body from these stresses.

One day Ms. Nichols appeared to me (JLG), complaining of increasingly painful abdominal cramps and headaches. Although first puzzled about what might have accounted for her worsening condition, our conversation soon centered on her frustration with her mother and sister who lived near her. Her mother and sister were both bitter and contemptuous about the new life choices Ms. Nichols had made during her therapy.

Upon visiting her mother and sister that week, Ms. Nichols noticed that she felt tense as soon as she walked through their front door, "like trying to push a wall down, but it won't go down." She felt they gave her "the cold treatment" with short, snippy answers to her questions and veiled insults in their comments. "It's a duty for a daughter to check on her mother. . . . It's like I'm trying to keep this family together, trying to do my part as a daughter and a sister. But in the back of my mind I know there's no family." She told how that she would try to relax at home after leaving her sister's home, but her mind would continue to dwell on the events of the visit, she would become more and more angry, and finally her head and abdomen would begin to ache. "My body is getting worse, instead of better as it had been in my therapy."

In questioning Ms. Nichols about her experience of the visit to her mother, we identified a dominant story that recruited her body into an emotional posture of bitter protest: "I'm trying to do my duty as a daughter and a sister, and I get the cold treatment. They treat me as though they want to see me upset or mad, because I am doing so well now and they don't have anybody to blame for their problems anymore." It was evident that the suction of this old story would draw her into double-bind communications with her family members. As a daughter she felt compelled by duty to visit her elderly, sick mother, but her experience of the visit was that of being attacked and punished, and there was no way in which the conflict could be discussed. Spoken inwardly over and over, these words would leave her more and more tormented, and her abdomen and head would begin to ache.

JLG: If you were to let yourself give up and follow wherever your body and feelings would take you, what would you do?

Ms. NICHOLS: Start crying . . . give up . . . I guess I would have a nervous breakdown.

JLG: What would the giving up be like? What exactly would you do that would represent your giving up?

Ms. NICHOLS: If I let go even a little bit, my mind would take me over . . . I would be at a breaking point . . . I would have to go into the hospital.

JLG: If you were to let go a little bit, what kinds of things would start filling your mind?

Ms. NICHOLS: My mind would just wander. My body would be doing things, but my mind would not be thinking. My mind would be unaware of what my body was doing. That is a frightening feeling.

She told how she became more and more tense when frightened that her mind and body would dissociate. She would try to slow down her mind from "going too fast for my body to keep up," repeatedly telling herself, "Slow down, Sarah. . . . Think. . . . Relax. . . . Your mind is going faster than your body. . . . You can't do it all at once." She could identify a "funny feeling" that signaled to her that her mind and body were about to dissociate.

I then asked if there were a complementary emotion within her body that signaled to her that her mind and body were working together, hand in hand:

MS. NICHOLS: When I get the feeling that I'm contented. I'm in control.

JLG: But exactly where in your body do you feel this contentment and control? .

MS. NICHOLS: In my stomach—my ulcer stops hurting. In the upper part of my body and my legs. My whole body feels relaxed.

JLG: And you can recognize that feeling in your body when it happens?

MS. NICHOLS: Yes.

JLG: Where were times and places in your life where you deeply felt this contentment?

MS. NICHOLS: [Reflecting] When I was home with my mother and we were living together . . . but I'm not there now . . . I felt that contentment when my children were little . . . but they are not little anymore.

JLG: If you flip back in your memories to each of these times, when you were home with your mother and when your children were little, and picture some of the scenes of what was happening then, just like you were watching a movie, which scenes bring the deepest contentment and control in your body?

MS. NICHOLS: [Pause] Well, my mother actually kept me under a lot of pressure. Everything had to be done perfectly. I feel more tense just imagining it.

JLG: And your children?

MS. NICHOLS: [Pause] I can see us sitting down, all together. I am reading stories. . . . Everyone listens.

JLG: Let yourself enter into the conversations, see the book, feel yourself speaking the words, hear your children's questions, notice the looks on their faces.

MS. NICHOLS: I feel content.

[She talked about fond remembrances when she and her children were all together, working together to survive as a single-parent family some- times, laughing and playing games together at other times.]

JLG: What you say is true, your children are gone now. But you can treat these stories with your children like pictures in an album that you can take out, look at, and feel the memories anytime you want, even if they are gone.

MS. NICHOLS: I can feel the contentment, but don't tell me to go back any further to when I was with my mother. That was when we were supposed to be a family, but we never were. I don't want to cross that line.

JLG: I'll bet that you know the verse in the Bible, "Whatsoever things are true, whatsoever things are pure, whatsoever things are just . . . whatsoever things are of good report. . . , think on these things"?

MS. NICHOLS: Yes. I do.

JLG: It's kind of like that. These stories about you and your children are stories of really being a family. You can choose which stories to think about.

Which stories would you like to choose? You can think about the stories that bring contentment, that bring healing, to your body. Would these be the stories that would bring contentment to your body?

Ms. NICHOLS: The stories of my real family—my mother, brothers, sister—are sad and tense times, so I push them behind. I think about me and my children. They are the good stories of my life.

After a bit more discussion, Ms. Nichols agreed that she could use her stories of her young children with her as a family as a way to find the contentment that protected her body. Her stories became for her another way that she could keep her disabling bodily symptoms at bay.

The steps taken by Ms. Nichols—identifying an emotional posture connected to symptom occurrence, binding self-narratives that anchor this emotional posture, a complementary emotional posture that precludes symptom occurrence, freeing self-narratives that anchor this protective emotional posture, then practicing ways to enter into the freeing self-narratives while avoiding the binding self-narratives—provide a readily available resource for care of the self that can be accessed at any time. A specific aspect of Ms. Nichols's situation that had rendered this avenue difficult to traverse had been her sense that her past was bundled as a unit—to remember times with her children would also mean remembering times from her own childhood in a family that was not a family. A distinction was offered ("You can choose which stories to think about—this is under your control") that, when appropriated by her as her own distinction, provided the empowerment needed to select only those stories that recruited her body into physiological states consistent with health.

An inward solution, such as that found by John and by Ms. Nichols, has been advocated in different forms for nearly two millennia by human beings, such as Boethius writing his *Consolation* from prison, who have sought inward answers for suffering when punishing, external circumstances are out of control (Buchanan & Oates, 1957). In our time, more than other clinicians, hypnotists have employed sensory imaging to reconfigure a patient's bodily state, thereby relieving a physical symptom, such as chronic pain, headaches, or asthma. Hypnotists commonly use guided imagery that emphasizes more static, primarily visual images in their work, such as: "Visualize the most pleasant and relaxing scene that you have ever experienced, perhaps a scene on the beach in summer, or walking through mountain forests, or a time when your family was happy and all together." Such generic instructions can be very effectively used by subjects already skilled in creating their own visual imagery or subjects who easily slip into a trance state. They are often less useful for subjects who are not so skilled.

By contrast, we do not seek a static scene, nor do we ask that the imagined image be pleasant and relaxing, although this is often the case. We seek instead to identify first a specific, idiosyncratic emotional posture out of which the symptom emerges and that is anchored by specific stories of lived experience. We use this emotional posture and its web of stories to guide us to a complementary emotional posture that can serve as an antidote for former's ill effects on the body. We then identify which stories of lived experience anchor this second, protective emotional posture. These are the self-narratives that can provide alternative stories into which a patient can deeply enter in order to find deliverance from his or her symptoms. These typically are very specific stories that we seek, special vignettes from remembered or fantasized social dramas. Of all the possibilities for working therapeutically with narratives in mind-body problems, we have perhaps relied most on this approach when symptoms have been chronic, sometimes stable for decades.

Helping a patient to access and use his or her own healing self-narratives to shield the body moves the struggle onto a different field—the body itself. A patient learns to take direct responsibility for his or her physiological body state. Instead of using narrative techniques to reshape its structure or to challenge its place in the discourse, a patient here learns how to deprive a binding self-narrative from having access to the body.

Instability of the emotional posture from which it emerges is a key point of vulnerability for a binding self-narrative. Unlike "ideas" or "beliefs," self-narratives seem to be able to dominate a person only when the body is set in a specific state of being. Like a hurricane whose power dissipates as quickly as it moves off warm gulf waters onto land, a binding self-narrative is destructive for the body only so long as it can draw strength from the specific emotional posture embodied in a specific physiological body state. For John, this physiological state was a poising of the body to receive expected rebuke and scorn for his failures. For Ms. Nichols, it was bitter rage held forcibly in check. When a patient selects a self-narrative, as did John and Ms. Nichols, that recruits the body into an incompatible physiological state, the destructive power of the binding self-narrative winds down into impotence.

Targeting Stories That Harm

It is one thing to enable a person to speak of his or her oppression; it is another to enable a person to speak when he or she has been only aware of the suffering, not of the oppression. The stories that are most malignant for the body are those that are not known as stories. They have become so much a part of the landscape of life that they are known by a patient as "this is the way life is."

Maurice Merleau-Ponty (1962) wrote about the totalizing power of moods. When I am elated, I do not see "elation"—I see an entire universe that is bright and blossoming. When I am depressed, I do not see "depression"—I see a somber and dark world everywhere I turn. In one moment, my entire world of experience is transformed into brightness; in another moment, it is transformed into darkness. Yet, I know directly only what has been transformed, not what was transformative. Similarly, self-narratives are totalizing in their transformation of experience, as in a dream when one loses memory that "this is a dream" and simply experiences events as they come—terrifying one night, delighting another night—as showing how the world, at that moment, "really is." Edward Bruner (1986, p. 144) has said, "Narratives are not only structures of meaning but structures of power as well." The power of a binding self-narrative resides in this kind of mystification of personal experience.

To aid the many patients suffering from mind-body problems, a way must be found first to distinguish a harmful self-narrative against the background of another account of one's life. In this step, a patient learns to see what afflicts. But a patient cannot be shown his or her experience; it must be discovered. The critical acts of the clinician, therefore, are not what the patient is told, how the patient is instructed, but what questions are asked. Questions with power are those that provide a wedge that can be driven between a binding self-narrative and the account of one's life within which it has become ensconced.

Here the work of a clinician is like that of a political tactician. A narrative that so constrains the body has become so familiar for a patient that he or she no longer knows it as only a narrative but also as a valid account of reality. The patient knows his or her suffering, but not the source from which it flows. The role of the clinician becomes that of one inciting to riot, of supplying contraband arms in the form of questions, metaphors, and stories that leave in the hands of the patient and family members a strong sense of personal choice and knowledge about how to meld learnings from everyday life into weapons fit to challenge the rule of symptoms that have governed their lives.

CHAPTER 7

Reauthoring Stories That Bind

INSTEAD OF BEING displaced or discarded, a binding self-narrative can be newly composed into a form that is benign. This recomposing, or reauthoring, changes either how the self-narrative is enacted in daily life or the text of the script that is enacted.

Dawn Tackett, for example, had been transferred to our hospital following a lengthy, failed hospitalization for unremitting headaches. During two stormy family meetings, she finally revealed a secret story that had tormented her: Dawn's father had abandoned the family without explanation while her mother had been pregnant with her. Haunted by the possibility that her approaching birth may have been to blame for his disappearance, Dawn had lived a depressed and troubled life. Six months earlier, her chronic vascular headaches had taken a malignant turn, worsening to such an extent that she began taking maximum doses of a multitude of headache medications, eventually ending in surgery and repeated hospitalizations. Dawn's secret was her new discovery: Using the computer resources and data bank access of her job, she had tracked down her father, learning that he lived in an adjoining state with a new marriage and other children. Her headaches had escalated in severity from this time of discovery, when she began struggling with her ambivalence about whether to go meet him and confront him.

For Dawn, the family meeting was more than an occasion in which she spoke openly her secret to her mother and sisters. She learned a piece of information she had never known: Contrary to her understanding that her father had disappeared with never a trace to his whereabouts, she learned from her mother that in fact he had checked back to make sure the new baby was okay. Evidently, there had been more to the story of his disappearance than she had been told.

For Dawn, this discovery was not trivial. Her story of her life underwent a rapid revision, from that of a woman whose entry into the world cost her family its husband and father, to that of a woman whose birth had been a secondary event in the disintegration of a marriage between her parents, and who, at least at some minimal level, had been shown concern by her father. Subsequently, Dawn's headaches began a dramatic descrecendo in frequency and intensity, with a concomitant cessation of aggressive medical treatment.

However important Dawn's speaking her dilemma to her family may have been, it seemed clear that this transformation of her life story was also a critical event in freeing her body from the constraints the old story had imposed. This transformation occurred spontaneously, purely by gathering the essential persons to talk and by facilitating the kind of conversation among them that fostered telling, hearing, and reflecting on important self-narratives.

Spontaneous transformations, such as that experienced by Dawn, suggest that deliberate, planned revision of self-narratives through literary craftsmanship may also open new possibilities for therapy of mind-body problems.

Performing Social Dramas with Binding Narratives

The important stories of our lives are those that are enacted by our bodies, more than those we simply tell or write for others. By way of analogy, thinking about a self-narrative as an enacted social drama better fits the clinical presentation of a mind-body problem than does speaking or writing a story. The anthropologist Victor Turner (1986) has insisted that a drama analogy is essential if we are to describe the richness of reality, experience, and expression as it is found in our social worlds. Turner has ascribed to persons the living out not of a life history but of a social drama in whose performance "what is" mingles subjunctively with "what could be" and "what ought to be." With many mind-body problems, the position of a patient is that of a deposed director, now become a mere actor in a play not of his or her choosing, performing a drama that tortures the body.

With Mr. Duquesnay, we discussed how problems in expression of storied experience can create binds that end in bodily symptoms. When a new social context was created in a therapy session that invited expression of his personal story, the telling proved to be healing. By contrast, we here describe how problems in the storying of experience can also create similar binds. The clinician's focus shifts away from studying the social context that governs expression to learning how a script is composed with which the patient performs his or her social drama. Assisted by the clinician, a patient and family can apply literary skills to identify, then to reauthor, those self-narratives whose performance has silenced expression of the body.

A drama analogy for understanding mind-body problems suggests two kinds of actions that can unbind a body: (1) A social drama can be restaged or recast; or (2) A script to be performed can be revised. In the former, a therapist asks questions that prompt change as to where in daily life a self-narrative is expressed or who will participate in it. In the latter, a therapist asks questions and suggests tasks that invite transformation of the old self-narrative into a new form or that encourage the authoring of a brand-new self-narrative.

Altering Contextual Markers to Transform a Binding Self-Narrative

Interpreting meaning is a task that human beings face when they need to understand the whole of something, whether a person, a situation, or an event. In seeking to understand a whole, people scan first for contextual markers, densely relevant signs that, taken together, direct us to the overall pattern we need to know.

Like punctuation marks that parse a mass of words into phrases, sentences, and paragraphs, contextual markers provide a short-cut to understanding what otherwise would require the examination of an overwhelming quantity of details at once. In human relationships, for example, a vital task is to know with which emotional posture one should approach the other (trusting, loving, controlling, threatening, detaching, scorning). How can one quickly grasp the whole of who the other is as a person, as well as his or her intentions? By reflex, our gaze goes to the face of the other and scans two key areas, the eyes and the mouth, in detail. The eyes, wide with wonder, glaring with rage, beady and ready to prey on, and the mouth, lips seductively pursed, drawn with tension, or warmly smiling a welcome, are critical contextual markers for our stance toward the other. Such powerful contextual markers appear to be phylogenetically determined to a great extent, as infants by the age of 5 months consistently show different emotional responses to different schematic faces with differently shaped mouths and eyes combined in different arrays (Wiener & Kagan, 1976).

Likewise, when we hear a narrative, we look for certain contextual markers that point to the pattern of the story, so that we can orient appropriately our experience. Consider a definition of narrative given by Theodore Sarbin

(1986, p. 3): "A symbolized account of actions of human beings that has a temporal dimension. The story has a beginning, a middle, and an ending. The story is held together by recognizable patterns of events called plots. Central to the plot structure are human predicaments and attempted resolutions," coupled with a comment by Donald Polkinghorne (1988, p. 18): "Narrative ordering makes individual events comprehensible by identifying the whole to which they contribute." These comments point to some of the contextual markers that we look for in hearing a narrative: its characters, setting, temporal punctuations (markers for beginning, middle, and ending), consciousness events (dilemmas, intentions, choices), and action events (what happens to the characters).

We use these markers to orient our personal experience to the narrative we hear, thereby creating our own narrative about the one heard, as we seek to grasp its core pattern, the minimal structure of which we term its plot. These contextual markers also show us where we can intervene if we seek to redirect the dramatic force of a narrative or to catalyze its transformation into a different kind of narrative.

Narrative reauthoring begins then by identifying the dominant narrative that is relevant to the mind-body problem. It is the ambiguities and unaccounted-for spaces within this narrative that provide possibilities for expanding the dominant narrative or for developing alternative narratives. No narrative account can fully state all that could be described about its subject. No narrative can include all events that plausibly could be included within its plot (Bruner, 1986a; Geertz, 1986). Every narrative conceivably could begin at a different point in time or could end sooner or later than the endpoint in the official version. There are thus manifold possibilites for alternative versions, all plausible, once the official or dominant narrative has been fully articulated.

Edward Bruner and Phyllis Gorfain (1984) have illustrated how this dialogical process works among stories on a national level. In writing about the Jewish story of the martyrs at Masada, Bruner and Gorfain showed how multiple differing accounts came to be told about the deaths of the 1,000 Jewish fighters who chose suicide rather than capture by the Romans since the brief, ancient account given by Josephus. Was Masada a defeat or a triumph? Did it prove the futility or the necessity of armed resistance against oppression? Was it the shame or the pride of a nation? As Bruner and Gorfain noted, the dominant version that has been told at different times in history has depended mainly on the use to which the telling was put, with different tellings sometimes having ends that conflicted—one telling, an argument for prayer instead of violence for redressing evil in the world; another telling, an argument to inspire confrontation of evil through heroic armed resistance; still another telling, a search to locate the version most stirring for the audience for a television spectacular.

But all the versions of the Masada story, even those offering contradictory interpretations of the meaning of the deaths, stand in relationship to one another. Secondary, alternative tellings of stories branch away from ambiguous or missing points in the story line of the official, or dominant, account. As Bruner and Gorfain (1984, p. 68) concluded, "The authoritative story as the dominant narrative provides the social matrix for dissident voices and secondary tellings. There may be a struggle over meaning, but one meaning is always taken with reference to the other. And all interpretations derive from the paradoxes, enigmas, and ambiguities inherent in the Masada story."

In our clinical work, we exploit these mutable features of a dominant narrative to help patients and families create more useful versions of stories that govern their bodies. Our fundamental intervention is the posing of questions that ask the patient and his or her family members to make sense out of the inconsistencies, ambiguities, paradoxes, and enigmas implicit in the dominant narrative. This request calls for patients and family members to create new meaning, thereby reauthoring or displacing the dominant narrative, in either case loosening the hold the story has on the body of the patient.

Toward this end, we have, to a great extent, drawn on clinical methods developed by Michael White and David Epston (Epston & White, 1992; White & Epston, 1990), two family therapists from Australia and New Zealand whose backgrounds in anthropology and sociology enabled them to recognize the practical possibilities for clinical treatment that lay in the arcane and academic scholarship of such anthropologists as Victor Turner, Edward Bruner, and Clifford Geertz, and such social scientists as Erving Goffman and Michel Foucault.

White and Epston (1990) note that a person typically presents to a clinician with a "problem-saturated" dominant narrative whose effect is to embody a problem within the person's self and body, all the while obscuring this influence from his or her awareness. Their strategy is first to identify and to externalize this dominant narrative, thereby objectifying and splitting it from the person's selfhood. Then gaps and spaces in the dominant narrative can be probed by inquiring about unique outcomes—life events that, although often unnoticed, contradict the dominant narrative. These unique outcomes can be expanded through deliberate, focused questioning into full-bodied narratives that can compete with the dominant narrative for space in the discourse.

We can briefly explicate White and Epston's approach by showing how it might be applied in therapy with Darlene, whose story was presented in chapter 2. Darlene's excruciating headaches arose out of an inward struggle against her fantasy to get a shotgun and blow away the head of her abusive father. When Darlene first arrived for therapy, she told only her problem-saturated story about failed treatments and a career as a headache-prone patient ("I am what they call a problem patient"). The binding narrative about her father lay unseen in the background.

In externalizing her problem, Darlene would be asked: "What are you like as a person when you are not dominated by the headaches? What about you do you value that the headaches keep other people from seeing? What is the history of how the headaches came to reside so prominently in your life?"

The headaches thereby become a "thing" external to who Darlene is as a person; Darlene becomes not a headache-prone, problem patient but a patient suffering under the oppression of unremitting headaches.

Subsequent questions, termed relative influence questions, would then map the political terrain between how much control Darlene held over the headaches versus how much control they held over her: "How many hours of the day do you find yourself dominated by the headaches? How many hours are you able to control them? What undermines your control of the headaches? What strengthens your ability to control them?"

Examination of what thoughts, ideas, or beliefs contributed most to the power of the headaches would bring to light the presence and power of the story about her father. Other questions would refine Darlene's awareness of the extent to which her life-style is organized by the headaches, how she has choices over whether or not to accept this influence, and how she can combat this influence by developing counterpractices, such as a refusal to be seduced into struggling with her fantasy. This strategy would thus challenge the dominant narrative about Darlene's headaches—a narrative about how she could only fight a determined, but losing, struggle against her headaches, much as she had only been able to fight a determined, but losing, struggle against her abusive father. Then shifting attention to the new story, numerous questions would be asked about unique outcomes in Darlene's experience—events in her experience that had gone unnoticed, because they had not fit well within her dominant narrative: "When were times when you would have expected headaches to occur, but, to your surprise, they did not? What was going on then? If you study carefully your headache-free days, what are differences that you notice about how you think, feel, or act on those days? What are personal qualities that you show on these days that reveal you to be the kind of person who can challenge the power of the headaches?" Accounts of these unique outcomes would then become the basis for a new narrative of Darlene's life that would protect against, not render her vulnerable to, headaches.

The thrust of White and Epston's clinical work is that of helping patients and family members become aware of how inculturated and institutionalized habits of perceiving, thinking, and acting have so shaped them that they have become symptom-bound. Once the covert influence of these social practices has been disclosed, the therapeutic work of deconstruction can then enable patient and family members to grasp previously unseen choices for shaping their lives in a more preferred manner. The work of therapy becomes a partnership between therapist, patient, and family members in designing effective counterpractices that create a life free of symptoms and more of his or her choosing. The clinical theory and methods originated by White and Epston have come to be called narrative therapy, or restorying therapy, as they are therapies within which the clinician consults to a patient and family in helping them to reauthor important self-narratives to disempower problems.

In a similar vein, we turn to the contextual markers of narratives, characters, setting, temporal markers, events, and the mutability they provide, in order to help patients to reauthor their social dramas in ways that free their bodies from binding dilemmas. Each of these contextual markers offers a perspective from which a patient's self-narrative can be reauthored.

Rescripting a Social Drama through Temporal Expansion

Starting a narrative a bit earlier or extending its endpoint further in time creates a turn-of-the-kaleidescope effect that instantly transforms the meaning of the narrative as a whole. Who has not had the rueful experience of arriving late for a movie and missing a critical opening scene, lacking which one entirely misinterprets the story presented during the next two hours of film? The same phenomenon can be put to therapeutic ends.

Reverend Jones, a 58-year-old minister, was referred for chest pain that his cardiologist attributed to anxiety, as treadmill testing and arteriography showed much less severe heart disease than would have been estimated from his frequent emergency room visits and repeated complaints of chest pain. During his interview, he spoke of the terror he felt when he sensed that he might be having a heart attack. In fact, on several occasions he had required emergency room treatment for authentic cardiac arrhythmias that could have been life threatening had no treatment been immediately available. Now, he felt panicky if traveling more than a few minutes away from an accessible emergency room.

Careful, moment-by-moment eliciting of his account of the minutes prior to and during his panic-filled chest pain revealed an important turn in his story. Reverend Jones spent nearly all his days immersed in a rich network of relationships he relished with family, friends, colleagues, parishioners, and his personal God. As he felt the grip of chest pain, he felt progressively more isolated from the presence of any person, including his God, as if death were closing in like darkness. His mind in fact would fill with images of doctors and nurses desperately pumping his chest, trying to resuscitate a dying man.

It was evident that Reverend Jones was repeatedly enacting his death scene down to the moment of his death. I (JLG) wondered to myself how his story could be expanded. I decided to ask what he would experience if he went even a bit further in time, to a moment beyond death. Surprised by the question, he paused, then told how once he did have a "near-death experience" in an emergency room in which he was entering a wonderful place of warmth and light and the presence of God. In this place of wonder, he felt no fear. Reconsidering his earlier chest pain and panic, we now talked about these moments of medical emergency as a liminal time, a brief segment of time between fear-free living on either side. During this liminal phase of medical emergency, "fear" had succeeded in separating Reverend Jones from his people and his God, a separation that he stated did not so much exist in reality as in that which he could then feel.

Thereafter, when chest pains started he concentrated on how he could sense with his body the felt presence of those he loved. Soon, he talked about how, even as his chest pain worsened, it was as if he could feel God's hand and fingers lightly on his chest. Although his cardiac pains regularly returned, his panic did not, and his frantic emergency room visits decreased markedly.

When a dominant, binding narrative repetitively starts or ends in unbearable trauma or doom, it is particularly helpful to press questions about how the story changes if started earlier or extended longer. When a victim shows posttraumatic symptoms, such as a woman who has been assaulted and raped, her narrative of the event is extended to end not with her attack but with her assailant's capture and her confronting him with her rage. A narrative of traumatic betrayal, when a lover left for another man, is extended past her humiliating dismissal to include the successes in life that followed her leaving and the realization of wisdom gained from having endured her loss. A man's story of having been cursed by birth in a poor, rural family with no resources or role model can be extended earlier to include stories of his forebears' faith, courage, and determination as they tilled the land—qualities he now prides in himself.

Rescripting a Social Drama by Recasting Its Characters

Adding or taking away characters from a drama powerfully alters interpretation of the story. Through questioning, a clinician can open possibilities either for recasting a social drama from the past or as it might occur in the future. A personal example shows the power of this transformation: When I was little, I (MEG) had very bad asthma. In the most severe episodes, my parents would have to drive me 150 miles to Memphis where I could be put under an oxygen tent and treated by a specialist in the big city hospital. These long drives were usually made in the wee hours of the morning following a sleepless night; yet, it is in remembering those nights that I find the deepest sense of comfort and peace today. These nights were not spent in my bed but in the big armchair in our living room with my father. I can still feel the texture of his seersucker robe as he held me, frightened and desperately wheezing, and began to calm me by reading from the *Reader's Digest Book of Children's Stories*. My breathing would begin to fall into rhythm with his measured breathing, which I felt as my head lay on his chest. The fear would melt away, and I finally began to rest. Once in Memphis, the sophisticated hospital treatments would be performed, but, for me, the essential help a sick child needed would always be the calm found in my father's lap.

It was a real jolt then when my own children would get sick, and I could not be as calm as my father. I needed to check the temperature, decide whether it was the right time to call the pediatrician, cancel what I could of the next day's schedule, and juggle the rest of my appointments with those of Griff's so we could figure out who could stay at home for which hours of the day. "Why can't I just be like Daddy was for me?" I despaired. "Instead of his calm, I am in a frenzy."

Then, one day while calling the pediatrician from my kitchen, it occurred to me that this was where my mother was when I was sick. She was in the kitchen busily making the telephone calls, getting me a room in the hospital, making arrangements for friends to keep my sisters, organizing the medicines, packing bags for all five of us, and trying to reach the doctor all at once. She was making the way smooth. As Daddy was carrying me, she was making a path. They complemented each other perfectly. His calm couldn't have been available to me without her activity. In the recasting of this life drama, my mother's behind-the-scenes role became central, forever changing the effect of that story on my life. My deep gratitude for her unseen involvement freed me to know that I was useful to my children in my frenzy and in my calm. I needed to be both, and I could be both.

Recasting a past drama can be accomplished through questions that either add characters, take some away, or expand the audience for its performance. This intervention played a role in the therapy of Tommy Bridges, the 9-year-old boy with a hacking cough, whose grandmother, Mrs. Lewis, would not leave his side (chapter 4).

We mentioned earlier that Mrs. Lewis told us about taking care of her daughter, Tommy's mother, as she slowly died from an undiagnosed infection as a complication of her multiple sclerosis. During her years of worry after her daughter's death, she wondered whether the outcome might have been different if she had been more vigilant and attentive. Within this story, her exquisite attentiveness and constant presence with Tommy made more sense. As I (MEG) talked with Mrs. Lewis, she began to relax and eventually considered taking a break away from Tommy. The introduction of her daughter into the drama as a new character was instrumental in permitting her shift into emotional postures of tranquility; as I asked more about her daughter, she told stories confirming that she had given her best to make her daughter's last months as good a life as they could be. Finally, I asked her, "What would your daughter say if she were here now?" "I reckon she'd say, 'Thank you, Mama. You did the best you could. I'm at peace now. It's good here.'"

MEG: If she saw you here with her son, Tommy . . . if she were here in this room with us, seeing you worry . . .

MRS. LEWIS: She'd kill me. "He's gonna be okay, Mama," she would say. And she'd for sure make me get some good sleep.

MEG: But that would mean leaving the room. Would she be worried about your leaving him with just the nursing staff to care for him?

MRS. LEWIS: No. It's a good bunch of nurses. She'd know that. She knew a lot about hospitals. No, she'd tell me to go home and rest.

MEG: But that would be so hard for you to do. What could she see from where she is now that you would listen to?

MRS. LEWIS: She can see us. She'd tell me, "You took good care of me, and you're taking real good care of Tommy. Now, you go get some rest. He'll be all right."

The introduction of another character—the daughter who had died—brought new possibilities into the drama being enacted, as we talked about her daughter's acceptance and appreciation of her mother and her understanding voice. Systemically, new possibilities appeared as the nurses and Mrs. Lewis approached each other with less suspicion and more understanding. In addition, the entry of her daughter into the conversation also released Mrs. Lewis from the kind of anxious watchfulness that, from the perspective of the pediatricians and nurses, was perpetuating the coughing.

Similarly, there can occur a recasting of characters for the future, depending on who is chosen to participate in solving the problem, who is left out, and who will constitute the audience. Recasting the future turns on determining which conversations need to take place: Who should be involved in which conversations at which times and for what purpose?

As discussed in chapter 5, we usually attempt in the beginning to gather all the persons engaged in language around a problem, the problem-organized system (Anderson & Goolishian, 1988), as our preferred unit for starting therapy. As the therapy progresses, however, we ask who should be included in the effort to solve the problem. Over time a problem-organized system evolves into a solution-organized system. Often, the two systems are not the same—solutions are sometimes more easily found when some of the participants originally in the middle of conversations about the problem are subsequently omitted. Sometimes, a solution cannot be found at all until a key person, or persons, is added to the conversation.

For example, Dawn Tackett was accompanied by her sisters, both bitterly angry, when she was transferred to our hospital for treatment of her headaches. They had agreed to the transfer only under duress, because her neurologist would discharge her from treatment otherwise. He had pursued every avenue in trying to relieve her headaches, but to no avail. When she now demanded narcotics to relieve her pain, he felt strongly that narcotic use would ultimately prove to be a serious error, failing to address the root cause of the headaches and exposing her to the risk of addiction.

The clinician called an initial family meeting, the first in which Dawn, her two sisters, and her mother sat together in the same room talking openly about her headaches. In this meeting, Dawn revealed how much she was upset by the constant arguing and fighting among her sisters and mother. She described herself as the peacemaker, the one always in the middle trying to get the others to make apologies to one another and to show appreciation for one another. She also hinted that there were private secrets that troubled her, but about which she could not speak.

Until this moment, her sisters had taken the lead in advocating aggressively on Dawn's behalf, angrily confronting medical clinicians whom they felt had failed to give to their sister the kind of care she needed, while also cajoling Dawn to follow their advice on dealing with her headaches. After this conversation, however, the sisters talked together and decided that Dawn needed her own space to work out her problems at her own speed. They convinced their mother to join them in backing away and offering help or advice to Dawn only when invited by her to do so. Henceforth, the therapy reorganized around Dawn and her husband as a couple as the usual therapeutic unit.

At the beginning of this therapy, Dawn's sisters and mother were a maelstrom of activity around her headaches. It was difficult to conceive of any way to work with her headaches without their participation. They thus were appropriately at the center of the problem-organized system gathered to begin the therapy. However, the therapeutic conversation began to show that their well-intended efforts were in fact presenting an obstacle to Dawn's resolving important, but presently unspeakable, dilemmas. In the recasting of Dawn's life drama for the future, the solution-organized system came to consist only of Dawn and her husband.

Rescripting a Social Drama by Changing Its Setting

Quite often, the problem-saturated description that a patient provides either claims itself to be a total description for all the patient's life or encapsulates the problem as isolated, cut off from other areas of life. "My whole life is one big headache"; "I am an epileptic"; "We are a diabetic family." Or, "When my Crohn's disease behaves itself, I am a happy person, and my life is great"; "My life is fine, except when these headaches start;" "There is nothing wrong anywhere else—these pseudoseizures come out of the blue."

The interpretations embodied in either description hide possible routes to solution. In the first case, they obscure evidence that in some situations the patient does know how to handle this kind of problem competently, and, in the second case, they obscure evidence that problem areas and non-problem areas of life are sufficiently interconnected that lessons learned in one area can be transferred to the other. To an extent, these limiting interpretations of experience hinge on what one takes to be the setting of the narrative constructed about the experience.

In the first case, a patient offers a narrative: "This is what the whole of what my life is about. . . ." A clinician then asks questions that inquire directly about areas of life that in fact have been resilient, unsullied by the problem's influence: "Are there any places or situations in your life where you find you do not have to be dominated by a man? What is different about these places? How have you managed to be in charge in these places?" These questions, by challenging the assumption that a narrative constructed out of life situations where failure occurred also provides a total description of life, alters the narrative by contracting its setting. Instead of a universal story, the narrative becomes a local story.

In the second case, the patient offers a narrative: "My life is discontinuous, with one part wonderful and the other part a mess." A clinician then asks questions about links between dilemmas in problem areas and similar dilemmas in non-problem areas: "Where else in the 'wonderful' part of your life have you ever felt in a bind dealing with an authoritarian man? How did you manage to escape entrapment in that situation? Where did you acquire the knowledge that enabled you to prevail?" This bridge building between problem domains and non-problem domains of experience can enable the patient to bring to the problem knowledge and skills that have operated effectively elsewhere. The narrative setting expands beyond the bounds of the problem domain to become, not a story of an isolated problem, but a story of struggle over a broad expanse of life, more intense in some places and less in others, with victory in some quarters but not yet in others.

We have learned through our clinical experiences that our patients and their family members can indeed prevail in their toughest life struggles by locating needed knowledge and skills already gained during everyday experiences. Useful questions are those that locate life experiences in which the particular dilemma of the therapy had been successfully worked out earlier at a different place, on a different scale, or at a different point in time. Through this dialogue, the setting for the narrative is extended beyond the domain of the problem.

The third session in the therapy of Tommy Bridges, the child with the hacking cough, illustrates a way in which a change of narrative setting can be accomplished.

I (MEG) could hear the cough as I approached the hospital room to make my third visit to Tommy and his grandmother, Mrs. Lewis. "I went to my sister's house and got a good night's sleep," she told me. "Tommy seems some better. I reckon it will take some time for him to get well." The pediatric pulmonologist had informed me though that the only reason she could find for his cough to continue was that it had become a learned habit. Tommy told me he could barely remember a time when he didn't have this cough. When I asked how much the cough troubled him, he guessed that he never went more than 2 minutes without coughing.

MEG: If we could work toward holding back the cough to every 5 minutes, instead of every 2, would that be of help?

TOMMY: Yes, ma'am. I could at least get a few deep breaths in then. But I've tried and tried, and I can't do it.

MEG: Maybe you would like to walk over to my office and talk. Okay, Tommy?

TOMMY: [Looking quite reluctant] You can just talk to my grandma.

MEG: Would you rather not talk now?

TOMMY: It's just that you talk too long. Grandma likes to talk, too, but I don't like long talks.

MEG: If we were to talk, about how long would be just right for you?

TOMMY: Well, about 20 or 25 minutes.

MEG: How about 20 minutes then? Will you hold the watch and let me know when we're out of time?

[A bit surprised, Tommy agreed. He took my watch and we started to walk to my office. I wondered what we could do in only 20 minutes. I noticed that as he became absorbed in the new sights and sounds, his cough continued, but the frequency decreased. The intervals now were more like 5 minutes than 2 minutes. I felt hopeful.]

MEG: Are you missing school much?

TOMMY: No, ma'am. I don't care much for school. Anyway my grandmother teaches me more than I could be learning these days at school.

MEG: But you must be missing your friends.

TOMMY: No, ma'am. They come over, and we all play Nintendo at my house. They know they won't catch my cough.

[About the time we reached my office, I again noticed my frustration building. Finally, I asked a question I should have asked in the beginning.]

MEG: How is the cough interfering with your life? What would you be doing if this cough weren't in your way?

TOMMY: Oh, I'd be playing baseball. I'd be at practice in the outfield, right now. My throwing arm is stronger now. Maybe I even would have been in the infield if I could've played this year.

MEG: Maybe so. And is being in the field the best for you or is batting the best?

TOMMY: Well, I reckon batting is the best when I hit it. I hit it good some of the time last year.

[Tommy was smiling and breathing more deeply and slowly. I paced my breathing to his and spoke softly.]

MEG: I like baseball. I wish you would tell me about your very best hit last year.

TOMMY: Okay. Well, we were playing the Green Team. They're real good. We're good, but they're real good. We had two outs already, and we needed to score some runs real bad. There was a guy on second and a guy on third.

[Tommy was taking deep breaths now without coughing. He had the far-away look in his eyes of a boy on the baseball diamond.]

TOMMY: I was up, and, you know, sometimes you just know you're gonna hit it? You know? Well, I knew I was. He threw me two balls, then the third one was mine.

MEG: [Still speaking softly and imaging the baseball game in my mind] Wow! Could you hear your team cheering? Could you hear the clapping?

TOMMY: No, I just heard the crack and I took off running. I went by first, and I looked and saw I could get to second, and I didn't even look then, I just ran on to third!

MEG: And then?

TOMMY: Oh, then my third base coach stopped me because the ball was coming to home plate. I got in on the next batter.

MEG: Could you hear your friends cheering then? I wonder if your Grandma got to see this?

[Tommy nodded, grinning widely, looking away. I imagined he was seeing her happy face in his mind.]

MEG: And what's that like when you hear the bat hit the ball?

TOMMY: I guess it's the best sound in the world.

MEG: You really love it, don't you? And you're pretty good at it, and getting better, it sounds. . . . You are also getting better at controlling your cough. I don't know how you did it, but while you were telling me about your triple, you completely stopped coughing! I guess we've been talking about that game for 12 whole minutes . . . and not one cough!

[Tommy was surprised, but he believed me.]

TOMMY: I don't know why it went away, but I can't make it stop. [Coughing again] I wish I could. [Obviously frustrated]

MEG: Tommy, there's something you know how to do at baseball, like "baseball breathing." When you bat and run around those bases, there's a kind of baseball breathing that keeps the cough away. Remember running . . . how you stretched out your legs and went by first, then by second, and got all the way to third? Can you remember it again?

[It was not hard for Tommy to go back to the diamond again. He focused, breathed deeply, and the cough subsided. He looked puzzled, but hopeful.]

MEG: You can do it. Just imagine you've heard the crack of the bat and are rounding the bases. The cough may pester you again sometimes, but you know the special way of baseball breathing, and this special place to go in your mind.

TOMMY: Maybe I can still play, too.

MEG: I imagine Dr. Sue would let you go pitch a few balls with the play therapist. Let's go talk to her now.

We walked back to Pediatrics. Tommy coughed only twice in that walk. He was quiet, happy, and thoughtful. We had only a few exchanges, mostly about baseball and the upcoming season. I talked with the nurses about his baseball life, and in a natural way they continued the conversation with him. Tommy was able to use his baseball skills, to put himself in the baseball setting, and to control his cough very quickly. He was discharged by the next afternoon. On his next return visit to the clinic, I learned that he had returned to school, still in control of his cough.

The setting of Tommy's narrative was extended from a circumscribed setting where he interacted with doctors, nurses, teachers, and his grandmother, to an expanded setting that included his exuberant play with his friends. His hacking cough thus became a local, rather than a universal, phenomenon. He was then able to import new bodily practices from untroubled to troubled areas of his life.

Rescripting a Social Drama by Altering the Selection of Events on Which Its Narrative Plot Is Constructed

A narrative is the fleshing out of a sequence of events impacted by, or having an impact on, the characters of the narrative. This sequence of events is its plot. The meaning of the narrative as a whole depends on which events are selected and how the meanings of those events are interpreted in composing a plot for the narrative. We are informed about which events to include by the characters' actions; we are informed about how to interpret these events through understanding the characters' motives and choices. Michael White (1988), drawing on the work of the cognitive psychologist Jerome Bruner, describes the sequence of selected events as providing a "landscape of action" and the interpretations of motive and choice as providing a "landscape of consciousness" for the narrative. We can reconstruct a dominant narrative by seeking alternative perspectives either for its landscape of action (which events are to be selected) or for its landscape of consciousness (new motives and choices are to be interpreted) or both. To further this aim, White (1992) advocates searching for unique outcomes out of which a more preferred narrative can be authored: "These landscape of action and landscape of conscious-ness questions are not simply questions about history. They are questions that historicize the unique outcome. And the re-authoring approach that I am describing here is not simply a process of pointing out positives. Instead, this approach actively engages persons in unravelling mysteries that the therapist can't solve."

In the following vignette, a husband initially presents his life story as one of irresponsibility and failure as a father and husband. This key self-narrative had organized not only his actions and habits but also those of the other family members, in a manner contributory to the paralysis that dis-abled his wife. In this initial interview, his act of encouraging his wife and children to participate in a family interview was identified as a unique out-come, around which a new history of the family began to be built.

Mrs. Mason was a 40-year-old woman, a homemaker, who had been referred to our medical center for paralysis of her arm and leg that had been diagnosed as a conversion symptom by our neurology service. As part of her psychiatric evaluation, she was asked to meet with our family therapy team together with her husband and her four children, Julia, age 8; Jackie, age 10; Nona, age 14; and Scott, age 17.

After an initial discussion about the neurologists' surprising diagnosis, Mr. Mason revealed that Julia had recently been molested by Nathan, a third cousin and church member who lived nearby and who was severely devel-opmentally disabled. This was an ongoing emotional trauma for all the fam-ily members, in part because they had not taken any effective action to remove Nathan from the community into a treatment program or protective custody, where he could not harm other children. Initially, they filed charges to have Nathan arrested but then dropped the charges under strong pressure from other family members and Mr. Mason's father, Reverend Mason, who was pastor of their small Baptist church. The stress of this irresolution had been so great that Mrs. Mason had asked for a divorce.

Although never discussed publicly in the community, it was in fact widely known that over many years Nathan had molested a large number of other children. His father, however, was a powerful social and political figure in the community and had always obstructed efforts to arrest or confine him. Nathan's father had argued convincingly that there were no adequate treat-ment programs for Nathan's problems and that Nathan would not be able to protect himself from harm in prison. He minimized the significance of Nathan's actions, because none of the victims had ever been physically injured.

Although Mr. Mason's father was in fact disturbed by Nathan's behavior, he expressed greater concern over the potential schism that could develop in their church if the church members began siding for or against jailing

Nathan. Reverend Mason strove to soothe his church members' angry feelings toward one another. He admonished his son not to make an issue over what had happened to Julia.

Mrs. Mason, however, felt an enormous burden of guilt, both for failing to protect her daughter and for her responsibility to protect other children who could be molested in the future. She had been having dreams that she interpreted as divine messages that this was indeed her responsibility. These presaged the onset of her inability to move.

MR. MASON: We thought we had an option to commit him to the mental hospital. They evaluated him as having the mental ability of a 10-year-old but said they didn't have treatment facilities for that kind of problem. Everyone got angry when we talked about filing criminal charges, and we didn't want to see him put in prison for the rest of his life either. We want to see him helped. But if there is not anything to do but file criminal charges. . . . I don't see why this responsibility has been put on my shoulders! Why didn't his father do anything? Why didn't Nathan's father or my father do anything? Nathan did this to my sisters. Nathan has been doing this for 25 years.

JLG: You mean, why your father didn't do anything when it touched your family?

MR. MASON: Yes. I imagine he just turned his back to it, like it wasn't there. "Leave it alone and it will go away." I have a lot of my father's attributes, I guess. But what I can't understand is that my parents knew about this all these years. And I am going to have to deal with it now. I've got to do something about it.

MRS. MASON: [Bitterly] No, you don't have to do anything about it. I will. That way you won't have any responsibility.

MR. MASON: No. It is my responsibility. I hate it, because I feel that I have done the same thing now that they did. And it has just about destroyed our marriage. . . .

JLG: Except that you have brought your family here, and you are talking about it. I don't get a picture of your parents as being people who would have come in.

MR. MASON: No. It wouldn't have been talked about. There wouldn't have been any discussion, much less with a stranger.

MRS. MASON: We've been married 15 years, and whenever I would ask them ` what was wrong with Nathan—he's not playing with a full deck, so to speak—they wouldn't even talk about what was wrong with him, like it was a hidden secret. Even talking about what was wrong with him physically or mentally.

JLG: So you've taken the step of breaking the rule of secrecy. You've taken the secret out of hiding.

MR. MASON: Oh, yeah! When we pressed charges, to make them have him evaluated and everything, my cousin—and this has happened to every one of his kids . . . Nathan has molested every one of his kids, and he knows the situation—he got mad at me, because he thought I was hurting the family. My father got mad . . . he knows there is a problem, but it is a situation of embarassment.

MRS. MASON: His cousin is more concerned with: "Don't embarrass me in the community." That is the bottom line with him.

MR. MASON: Yeah.

JLG: Julia, this happened with you. Did it happen with you, Nona?

NONA: He messed with me when I was a little kid.

MR. MASON: See, we didn't know about that until it happened with Julia.

JLG: I guess this is a dilemma. This is something very hard to talk about. And I think that there is in many families a pressure just to cover it over. You know that happens a lot. [To the girls] Would you prefer that your father speak out and break the secrecy, or would you prefer that he cover it over, as his father did?

JULIA: What I feel is that Nathan should serve time and also get help. And I think Dad needs to press charges. Because, what if he is doing it to somebody right now?

JLG: So you would prefer that your father speak out, rather than taking the path of his father?

JULIA: Yes. Because Grandpa knew what he did and let it go by. Uncle William [Nathan's father] knew what he did and let it go by. But if they keep on letting it go by, he will keep on and keep on and keep on.

JLG: How about you, Nona? Would you prefer that your father break the secrecy and speak out, or would you prefer that your father cover it over like his father did?

NONA: I would prefer that he speak out and tell everyone and get Nathan in jail or prison or somewhere. And get him help, because he does need it.

JLG: It sounds like your father is very different from his father.

Rather than providing evidence that Mr. Mason was of similar character as his father, his speaking out in therapy and his heeding his wife and daughters became evidence—as unique outcomes—that he was a man of courage instead. In subsequent sessions, questions were asked that expanded a new story of Mr. Mason's life and a new story of the family: Was this the first time he had stood with courage, or might there in fact have been other occasions? What life experiences had provided him with the wisdom and strength of character to act, rather than to cower, during this crisis? Had Mrs. Mason perhaps noted these distinctions between Mr. Mason and his father during previous decisions during crises? If his daughters were ever to face this kind of terrible dilemma with their children, how would he wish them to make a choice? If Mr. Mason were to continue to model these kinds of choices for his children as years go by, what kind of character traits would he anticipate they might develop through modeling their father?

Along a landscape of consciousness and a landscape of action, these questions and the creative reflection they prompted slowly built a new story of the Mason family wherein Mrs. Mason's body remained strong.

Inferring a New Narrative from the Body's Expression

Sometimes, a narrative hides so well that all we can find are its tracks on the patient's body. But by studying carefully the traces left, we can sometimes reconstruct a plausible narrative as it might have existed, and, by reworking this prototype, rework the impact the original narrative left on the patient's body. Most often, this is the case when there historically has been a specific catastrophic trauma whose memory is presently dissociated from everyday awareness, but whose impact continues to be felt in painful or disabling somatic symptoms. Pains, numbness, menstrual symptoms, weakness, vomiting, nonepileptic seizures, dizziness, and hypersensitivity to specific kinds of sensations are common adult sequelae of childhood physical or sexual abuse and of other forms of posttraumatic stress disorder. A therapy with Caleb shows how therapeutically powerful inferred narrative can be constructed.

Caleb might have kept on enduring forever the episodes of excruciating pain and fear that jolted him out of his sleep. They didn't happen often, and he had learned early in life not to be a "troublemaker." But he was worried. He was engaged and worried about what these problems might do to his marriage. He was a therapist-in-training and worried about what any unresolved issues might do to his work with his own clients.

He began to tell me about the fear and revulsion he felt around his uncle, about his mother's relating the story of her own sexual abuse, and the history of sexual abuse in their family. Now Caleb's pain, nightmares, and the distracting bodily sensations he experienced as he sat with his sexually abused clients prodded him to wonder if "something may have happened" to him. "I think it may have happened," he said. "If it did, then I need to know—but I can't remember anything specific. Maybe it didn't happen, or maybe what did happen was not as big a deal as I think. What I really, really hope is that I can see you, and you will tell me that nothing happened. Then, I can put this behind me, once and for all."

Then he told about the frequent terrifying experience of his nightmares: He would awaken, not clearly remembering the nightmare but feeling an awful visceral pain. He would be startled by the fear that someone was standing over him, watching him with a predatory stare. Although he knew no one was there, he felt compelled in his darkened room to get up, turn on the lights, and check under the bed and in the closets before he could rest. He felt humiliated to be doing this. His head hung in shame, and he drew his arms and legs close to his body as he told me quietly, "And the pain. It's difficult for me to tell you about it. It's a terrible pressure that won't go away. It scares me a lot. I feel like I want to run, but I have to be completely still and wait for it to stop. I try to push it away, but I can't. I just have to lie there and wait."

First, we worked with creating safety in the night. He was a deeply spiritual man and decided to image God with him as the understanding father he needed to help him to turn on the lights and check the closets, accepting Caleb's fear and giving him courage.

Then we talked softly for a long while about where the path might lead for his speaking about the sexual abuse if it had happened, where the path might lead if he knew it happened but did not speak out, and where the path might lead if he were never to know but were to wonder aloud about it with his family members. Each of these paths was fraught with risks, but he felt in the end that the most liberating path would be the one of knowing the truth and speaking it as honestly as he could. He wondered, however, if he were making "something out of nothing."

"Surely, it sounds as if there may have been some terrible experience that your body can remember. The other things you say sound as if it's even likely that you were abused. And you may never remember, but you are beginning to remember your nightmares. If you can be in a safe place, in the daytime, when your fiancée and best friend know what you are about, maybe you can begin to write—not your memory, but what you think might have happened, the best you can piece it together. We will look together, not taking it as truth, but as a starting place, as the wondering aloud that you wish you could do with your family."

In the weeks that followed, Caleb did begin to wonder aloud. Surrounded by the love of his fiancée and of his God, and encouraged by his mother and his friends, his vagueness turned to clarity about the sexual abuse his uncle had perpetrated. The pain that had paralyzed him became his wise memory. It troubled him again a few times, but, he said, "It doesn't have the power it used to have. I don't have to stay still and stay scared." Near the end of our work, after he had confronted the uncle, I asked him, as I had in each session, what he felt in his body. "I can breathe," he said. "I can move, and I can breathe."

Problems and Pitfalls in Reauthoring
Self-Narratives

We have taught these clinical methods to a variety of mental health clinicians in recent years. Some difficulties in learning occur more commonly than others.

Probably, the most common source of error, at least for clinicians trained in traditional medical and graduate schools, is to forget that the patient and family members are the bona fide authors of their new story; the clinician serves only as a consultant. Meaning expands, and bodies are freed from symptoms by building on the stories patients bring, not the professional stories clinicians offer. Initially, this understanding is difficult for novice clinicians, because it contradicts the doctrine of professional education that would have the clinician, as expert in and bestower of scientific knowledge, specify which story needs reauthoring and what the revision should look like.

Other closely related errors are made by assuming too much. It is easy for a less experienced clinician to assume automatically what patients and family members would prefer ("Of course, no one would want that!") when in fact that is exactly what the patient would select within a forced choice. The story of Frances in chapter 3 provides a poignant example of such a surprise, when, to the clinician's amazement, her sisters understood that Frances might choose to die rather than confront their mother with the truth.

As a natural consequence of this following-the-patient posture, a clinician primarily asks questions, rather than makes declarative statements. Such questions need to be made from a "not-knowing" position of therapeutic noncertainty, but this mode of interviewing feels counterintuitive to clinicians traditionally trained.

It is also difficult for many psychodynamically trained clinicians to avoid making interpretations. It is a central tenet of this approach that there is no interpretation to be made when one authentically accepts the patient's right to authorship of his or her story. Yet, when clinicians are trained to hear patients' stories "with a third ear," it becomes automatic to orient themselves primarily to what they interpret the patient to mean, rather than what the patient in fact is saying.

Finally, novice clinicians often fail to identify carefully enough those self-narratives that are tightly connected to the symptom via its associated emotional posture. It is easy to focus mistakenly on an easily accessible, but superficial, story that holds little power for coordinating states of the body. With Frances, for example, little would have been accomplished by attempting to work solely with the story of her chronic struggle with bulimia, rather than her story of abuse as a child.

It is our impression that most of these problems and pitfalls are consequent to habits of communicating with patients that are learned in the trade schools of medicine and psychology. These habits ill serve patients and families who are objectified and silenced by them.

CHAPTER 8

Seeking Competence in Language Skills

SKILL FOR A THERAPIST resides in knowing how to use language to build relationships, to create conversations, and to catalyze meaning that can serve as a new solution for an old problem. How can a clinician gain the competence to use language to solve mind-body problems?

There are two sets of language skills in which expertise is especially needed if a clinician is to conduct therapy productively. The first is skill in establishing optimal conditions for the kind of reflection that generates new meaning; the second is skill in crafting questions that facilitate therapeutic change. With these skills a clinician hopes not only for patients and families to find good answers for their current problems, but also that they will learn how to ask fruitful questions that bring answers to future problems without the intervention of a professional.

The Training Dilemma

The task of learning how to use language effectively in human relationships is daunting for many clinicians in training. Trainees bring years of experiences with practicing and drilling in classrooms and on athletic fields when striving to learn new skills. Professional education frequently is little different in its emphasis on the rote learning of technical skills. During my last year of medical school, for example, I (JLG) practiced daily my sutures and surgeon's knots on sows' ears brought home from the butcher. As a nursing student, I (MEG) repeatedly wrote nursing care plans that came to be less individualized and more standardized with each patient I nursed. Psychology graduate students repeatedly administer intelligence tests to volunteers until the reliability of their testing is sure. Every professional discipline drills its trainees in its particular technology, so that the same therapeutic action can be performed with greater and greater reliability on one patient or client after another.

So how does one master skills needed for using language to influence healing of the body? Is there a language technology in which trainees can hone their skills with drills and exercises? This question has been exhaustively examined by the hermeneutic philosophers. "There is no such thing," Gadamer concluded, "as a method of learning to ask questions, of learning to see what needs to be questioned" (Fiumara, 1990, p. 49). The verbal dance between clinician and patient is simply too fluid and too polymorphous for any standardized routine or set of rules to prescribe ahead of time what to say in a conversation. To program precisely the asking of questions in therapy is to invite angry confusion or compliant boredom from patients and family members who appropriately feel misunderstood.

Yet, there exist pressures to create clinical practices that would function as if they were rules. Society's agenda in the 1990s is an economic one of moving a person from "patient" status to "nonpatient" status as quickly and as cheaply as possible, so much so that concern over reducing suffering is often secondary in importance.

We have looked for a middle ground in training that lies somewhere between creating a "technology of language" and renouncing any consistent principles that guide how language can be best used in clinical practice. Although they are not as precise as rules or laws, we can propose more or less reliable guidelines for the use of language. These guidelines are reliable only to the extent that we as clinicians share with each other language practices drawn from biological similarities as talking mammals, and social similarities as partakers of a common culture. They are heuristics that have enough leeway in precise applications that each can be organized around the uniqueness of the person of the clinician and the conversation and relationship within which it is applied. As Tom Andersen has said, such guidelines "might be regarded as a sort of scaffold, as they can be set in many ways and are transitional" (Andersen, 1991, p. 42).

Crafting Useful Questions

Our therapeutic approach mainly rests on the asking of questions, instead of making instructive statements. It is easier to avoid being "too unusual" with questions than with declarative statements (Andersen, 1991, p. 34). Every question does have a horizon of meaning. That is, every question has a finite set of answers that are potentially acceptable, giving each question a specific direction of influence. But questions, as half-statements (Gadamer, 1976), influence less than do declarative statements and are therefore less likely to be experienced as oppressive. Consider the difference between the following two utterances spoken to a mother and her daughter with anorexia during a family meeting: (1) "Daughters with anorexia need less emotional involvement with their mothers"; and (2) "What kinds of times together and conversations between you seem to strengthen you against the influence of anorexia, and what kinds seem to leave you more vulnerable?" It is apparent that the latter utterance conveys less a sense of certainty by the speaker, leaving more space for the mother and daughter to express how they experience their individual relationship.

Why is it that some questions are consistently more useful than others? Some questions seem to be effective, because they actively invite curiosity or openness, rather than prompting alarm or protest. Others appear to be effective primarily because the clinician entered an emotional posture of tranquility before asking the question.

A question asked from an emotional posture that is either disaffiliative toward or specifying of the other constricts possibilities for new meaning or creative actions by the other. Such emotional postures can be either disaffiliative emotional postures, such as scorning, belittling, or indignant, or affiliative, yet disempowering, emotional postures, such as condescending, paternalistic, or indulging. Along the same lines, Lynn Hoffman (1985) has offered the dictum that nobody changes under a negative connotation—at least not easily. Conversely, a question asked within affiliative and empowering emotional postures, such as respectful, reverent, curious, or open postures, generates new meanings and actions that are likely to be therapeutic.* The meaning of a question asked in therapy seems to depend as much, or more, on the emotional posture within which it is asked as it does on its semantic structure.

The crafting of questions that engender therapeutic change has been a major contribution of family therapy to the mental health disciplines (Slovik & Griffith, 1992). The Milan team in 1980 used cybernetic theory to conceptualize "circular questions" to track interpersonal processes in families. Their work was systematized and expanded by Peggy Penn at the Ackerman Institute (1982, 1985) and Karl Tomm in Calgary (1987a, 1987b, 1988). A new generation of strategic therapists at the Brief Therapy Center in Milwaukee (De

*These ideas about the therapist's emotional postures leading to types of questions that close or open patients' possibilities for new meanings and action is akin to the ideas presented by Karl Tomm (1990). Tomm plots a therapist's behaviors along a continuum that runs between therapeutic love (opening options) and therapeutic violence (closing options).

Shazer, 1985; Lipchik, 1988) used constructivist theory to design question-sthat focused on potential solutions, rather than the problem to be solved. In Australia and New Zealand, Michael White (1986, 1987, 1988) and David Epston (1986; Barlow, Epston, Murphy, O'Flaherty, & Webster, 1987), drew on critical theory, social constructionism, and narrative theory to create sequences of questions that empower persons to reauthor the guiding narratives of their lives and, thereby, their selves.

These clinicians each adopted a specific clinical theory that inspired the types of questions that embodied the theory. Most centered on the semantic structure of the questions. We have relied on each of these contributions to derive useful questions for pursuing mind-body problems. However, we place a primary emphasis on asking questions from within emotional postures of tranquility, such as curiosity, respect, and openness. Further, we have studied how certain questions can open access to emotional postures of tranquility.

The work of the Tromso team in Norway illustrates nicely the value in first finding an emotional posture of tranquility before crafting a question. The Tromso clinicians often ask quite simple questions. ("What have you been thinking about?" "What do you want to do in this session? Might there be other possibilities?" "Do you have any comments on what has been said?") in contrast to the complex questions intricately designed by other clinicians. Yet, those who have personally witnessed the clinical work of the Tromso clinicians have been struck by its therapeutic power, evidently due to their characteristic warm acceptance, interest, and openness (Tjersland, 1990).

Because the emotional posture of the therapist is critical for shaping the evolution of the therapeutic conversation, the clinician's own inner questioning of self during therapy is as important as the questioning of the patient and family members. For example, a clinician who wonders about and reflects on what questions could be asked, yet have not yet been asked, tends naturally to drift into emotional postures of curiosity and openness that foster similar emotional postures in the patient and family members. These "questions not yet asked" provide an important tool for enabling a clinician to remain within emotional postures conducive to a therapeutic relationship (Andersen, 1991, p. 35).

Some questions are particularly effective, because their semantic content invites emotional postures of tranquility. These include questions that:

1.) Juxtapose meaning in unexpected ways: "If you were to show to yourself the same care and concern that you have shown to the children in your classroom, how do you suppose your Crohn's disease would experience the difference?"

2.) Shift attention to regions of life experience that have been neglected or overlooked: "If there ever were times when you were in a relationship with a man and experienced no sign of fear in your body, when might that have been?"

3.) Introduce new cognitive frames for organizing experience: "When you are enjoying solitude and when you are lonely, what do you feel in your body that tells you it is one or the other?"

4.) Open space for a range of possible answers, hence space for the unexpected creativity of the patient: "You said that you feel deep bitterness toward your sister. If you draw close to those words, 'deep bitterness,' what exactly do you taste? What do you see? How does your body experience this tasting and seeing?"

Finally, some questions seem to have therapeutic efficacy, because they counter culturewide social practices that are contributory to generating and perpetuating mind-body problems. These include:

1.) Questions countering cultural practices that consistently direct attention away from certain domains of experience, hence leaving them unexamined (Andersen, 1991): "If you looked over all the different things that you do in order to please your children, which ones would your body most protest if it were to voice an opinion?"

2.) Questions that facilitate a shift to an alternative epistemological position (Griffith & Griffith, 1992b). There are three epistemological positions in any conversation: addressing the other, being addressed by the other, and listening to others converse (the reflecting position). Remaining habitually in one position limits options available for creative problem solving. It is often the case, however, that the rigidity of an entrenched problem is isomorphic with rigidity in the intrapersonal discourse of the person having the problem. That is, being stuck in a problem is often experienced inwardly as a running conversation from a single epistemological position, even though the need is great for as many available options and perspectives as is possible.

For example, Joanna was a young woman who would become suicidally depressed with self-recriminations of "You don't really want to get better. You are nothing but a burden. They would be better off without you." Under these self-recriminations, Joanna only experienced herself from an under-the-gaze, being-addressed epistemological position. One line of questions in her therapy sought to enable Joanna to view her situation from other epistemological positions:

1.) Addressing position: "If you were a fairy whispering these words into Joanna's thoughts—'You don't really want to get better. You are nothing but a burden. They would be better off without you.'—what would you be noticing about Joanna that would prompt you to say these words? As you spoke these words, what emotion toward Joanna would you be experiencing? What would be your intent; that is, what would you hope might happen by speaking these words? Would you be wishing goodness or badness for Joanna by whispering these words into her thoughts?"

2.) Reflecting position: "If you could be a fly on the wall observing Joanna during one of her moments of black depression, what might you see that she would not be able to see? What would you notice about the conversation between Joanna and the voice inside her? Could you see a way for her to use this inner dialogue creatively to help her depression?"

3.) Questions that are asked out of a nondominant tradition: These include questions about a bodily symptom asked from a political, economic, moral, religious, or cultural frame of reference: "When you feel the pressure of the idea that whenever women are not actively serving their families they are a burden to them, how does your mindfulness of your body change? Are you more attentive or less when it signals distress?"

4.) Questions that create a conversation in which the patient's body has a voice, especially when the body previously has had no voice: This specifically counters social practices that demand a silencing of spontaneous bodily expression in order to preserve the status quo in social relationships. "When your stomach began hurting while talking to your husband, what would your stomach have said if it were to have had a voice?"

The Reflecting Position

A reflecting position is a listening position. In its most fundamental aspect, it is a place in a conversation where one can listen to others talk without feeling compelled to respond to what is heard, or listen freely to one's inner talk without feeling compelled to relegate it to total secrecy or total exposure.

Although some clinicians over the years have conducted conversations during therapy sessions, either between cotherapists or between a therapist and observation team members, such conversations usually were either instructive or manipulative in intent. That is, the conversations were staged either to teach the patient and family or to trigger a desired behavioral change in the family system. It was not until the work of Tom Andersen and his colleagues in Tromso, Norway, (1987b, 1991, 1992) that the intent of an intrasession conversation among therapists came to be nothing other than creating a context that would invite the listening patient and family members to create new meaning.

With a traditional reflecting team consultation, a team of observers and the clinician-patient-family switch places at some point during the session, so that the latter can watch and listen to the team discuss the problem, as the team has thus far witnessed it. The reflecting team and clinician-patient-family then switch back, so that the patient and family members can comment on the team's discussion (Andersen, 1987b, 1991). There are a variety of possible permutations that also embody a reflecting position—for example, the reflecting team can interview the therapist about the session in front of the patient, or the reflecting team can come into the therapy room to provide the consultation discussion rather than switching rooms (Andersen, 1991).

The rules of procedure for working in therapy with the reflecting position are simple and straightforward (Andersen, 1992):

1.) The consultant clinician or team bases their comments on the utterances spoken within that specific session, not using information drawn from some other source, such as information from the medical chart or reports made by other hospital staff. ("When I heard. . . " or "When I saw . . . I had this idea") (Andersen, 1992, p. 60).

2.) Comments offered are made tentatively. ("Maybe you heard something else, but I heard. . . ") (Andersen, 1992, p. 60). This provides the widest possible latitude for the patient's and family members' wonderings.

3.) Critical, scorning, belittling, or shaming comments are avoided. Anyone who has accidentally overhead oneself discussed in a derogatory manner in another conversation knows the power of the reflecting position for magnifying hurt. Statements such as: "It appears that Mr. J. depends on his headaches to gain his wife's attention" or "The mother doesn't give her daughter the space she needs in order to grow up" are pathologizing statements that would slam shut the door to reflective listening, rather than opening it (Andersen, 1992).

4.) Short of being discourteous, the reflecting team members maintain eye contact and talk among themselves, rather than opening the conversation to include the patient or family members. If the patient or family members enter into the discussion, they usually leave the reflecting position (Andersen, 1992).

5.) Comments are mostly made within a "both/and" framework, rather than "either/or," so that the range of possible solutions can expand. "I wondered whether there might be a way that each person in the family could have a desired amount of privacy, yet, the family would remain a close family?" "I noticed that Judy showed affection toward her mother and also asserted her position firmly" (Andersen, 1992).

6.) Telling what was noticed and relating that to the consultants' thoughts, images, or imaginings are more emphasized than evaluating, judging, or explaining what was observed. A statement such as, "I heard Judy say 'I want to feel that I am my own person' three times during the session. I wondered what memories came to mind for each of her parents as they recalled their teenage years" would be preferred to a more interpretive, evaluative statement such as "Judy is showing us that she is determined to establish her autonomy and independence within the family."

These guidelines make transparent the cognitive processes of clinicians, what they notice and how they think. They also create a democratic structure for therapy, in which one perspective cannot dominate simply because it is loudest or most intense (Hoffman, 1992). The structure enables the patient and family members to observe respectful speaking, listening, and reflecting modeled by the clinicians. Such conversations may be rarely experienced in daily life.

In chapter 7, we told the story of Mrs. Mason, the homemaker who was referred for conversion paralysis. The success of the initial session with the family was facilitated by a reflecting consultation. The family members had been discussing their dilemma, whether to overlook the criminality of Nathan's sexual abuse of their daughter out of loyalty and respect for Mr. Mason's father, or whether to press criminal charges against Nathan out of loyalty and respect for their own children.

Julia and Nona, who had been molested, had each expressed strong convictions that their father should press criminal charges against Nathan.

JLG: How about you, Nona? Would you prefer that your father break the secrecy and speak out, or would you prefer that you father cover it over like his father did?

NONA: I would prefer that he speak out and tell everyone and get Nathan in jail or prison or somewhere. And get him help, because he does need it.

JLG: It sounds like your father is very different from his father. [Pause] This might be a good time to get some thoughts from some of our team. What we often do is to first talk together some, then let the team of clinicians who are observing come in and share some of their ideas.

[The reflecting team members, Melissa (MEG) and psychiatry resident Bill Turner (BT), enter the therapy room and seat themselves in a circle in front of the family members]

MEG: I was most moved by the family breaking the secrecy. It seems like an incredibly hard thing to do, especially with such a large, extended family that for years has protected Nathan from the consequences of his actions. . . . I am not sure what the steps will be from here. Mr. Mason sounds like he does want to do something. . . . One thing that I wondered about—Mr. Mason had mentioned that all the family members were strong members of their church—I wondered what their conversations with God had been like about this. I wondered about that. It seems that Mr. Mason, like Julia, wants for all of them to receive justice and compassion and protection, not only for his own daughter, but also for anyone else who could be a potential victim of Nathan's.

BT: I was impressed that they were all so unified with the same idea of protection for others, and not just for themselves. They do seem to be unified in the idea that something needs to be done, not so much for blaming but for making things safer for the future.

MEG: There seemed to a really strong theme of openness. When the girls were talking about their lives with their friends, they said they liked to talk, to talk about everything. And Mr. Mason said, "We need to have this meeting. We need to talk about things." Mrs. Mason and Nona told how Mrs. Mason's illness has gotten in the way of their being able to talk as a mother and daughter the way they would want to be able to talk with each other. It seemed that there is a strong yearning for openness and talking.

BT: Mrs. Mason said she wanted to find out what is wrong. She wants to find out why she became paralyzed. She is not satisfied simply to be treated for the symptom. She wants to get down to the root of the problem. . . . I wonder how solving this problem of Nathan will affect her level of stress at home?

MEG: I was curious to know in relation to her paralysis—listening to Mrs. Mason tell about sitting on the floor at home and crying and feeling like she was not in control of her life—I wondered if in this conversation she felt more in control of her life. I wondered if talking in this way put the Masons more in control of their life as a family. I wondered what they will think about after this. It seems to me that they are going into uncharted territory. Mr. and Mrs. Mason are creating a new, different, more open kind of life for their family than they knew when they were growing up as children. I thought of people going out into a new land, clearing out the brambles and moving forward.

[The reflecting team members return to their observation room.]

MR. MASON: Martha became paralyzed last week. Then, I was in the hospital until Thursday. When I got out, Martha told me she wanted a divorce. She said she needed to get control over her life. She felt like she didn't have any control over it. I know she also felt trapped in our marriage. She felt I had been more considerate and respectful of other people's feelings and wishes than I had been for her and our family. I realized then that I had made some serious mistakes in the marriage. But I love her. [Begins weeping] Perhaps her inability to walk is a lot my responsibility, or even mostly mine. [Weeps]

JLG: It sounds as if there are terrible dilemmas in the family having to do with responsibility. [To Mrs. Mason] Like in your dream, feeling responsible for the children who might yet be harmed in the future. [To Mr. Mason] And your feeling here that "maybe I'm responsible for the problems in the marriage." Terrible dilemmas about responsibility. [Silence]

One thing I believe is that it is important to respect dilemmas for what they are. Usually, they are these places in life where we feel, "I've got two choices. But either choice I take is the wrong thing to do." They can be really sticky to deal with. I believe it simply is important to respect the difficulty. When we first started talking, we talked about what the paralysis was like, then about what role worry might play in causing it, then about what happened to Nona, then the guilt and responsibility about whether to act or not to act. . . . It sounds as if it comes down to this: To take action with Nathan that would protect the children would be experienced by your family as betraying and shaming them. That is a terrible dilemma to be in, but to what extent do each of you believe that dealing with this would be the starting place for doing something that would keep Mrs. Mason's body strong?

JULIA: I believe what would help Mama and her body is that something be done about Nathan. I think that would take a lot of pressure off her. And I think my parents need to see a marriage counselor and sit down and tell their true feelings and work things out, because the last thing they need is a divorce.

JLG: Would you all agree with Julia?

MRS. MASON: I don't know if that is what is causing the trouble walking. But I would feel better.

JLG: I wonder. What would be the next step to take toward working out what to do?

MR. MASON: I have enough evidence to press criminal charges. I want to use that to try to get him into some kind of treatment program. But there isn't any available.

JLG: What is the difference that you see between yourself as a person and your father?

MR. MASON: I've been a visionary, but I look at things realistically—there are real problems, there are real situations that have to be dealt with. I have a tendency not to go through with things. But this is a situation that has got to be dealt with. [Pause] I love my children. I certainly don't want them ever to grow up and to think that something happened, and I didn't do something to protect them. I want to be a good father. And I want them to always think of me as a good father. I love my father, and I think of him highly, but I think in some respects, he wasn't a very good father. [Begins to weep]

JLG: That is an enormous difference.

During the reflecting team consultation, team members spoke about how moved they were that Mr. Mason would break with his family rules and traditions to embrace openness, justice, and protection for his children and those in other families. Prior to the reflecting team consultation, the family had acknowledged for the first time the dark secrets that haunted them: Both daughters had been sexually abused, and the perpetrator still lived unrestrained in the community, protected by his father, a powerful patriarch who minimized the abuse. But the consultation immediately brought forth a secret even more threatening to the family, a threat of the parents divorcing. The threat of divorce and a plan to evade it were then discussed, respectfully and thoughtfully, by all present.

The unspeakable binds that often characterize mind-body problems forbid discussing in everyday conversations the kinds of dilemmas that create these binds. A reflecting team consultation can establish a dialogical space where the unspeakable can be spoken (Andersen, 1991; Griffith & Griffith, 1992b). This conclusion was supported by an empirical study of patients presenting a somatic symptom. We utilized the Structural Analysis of Social Behavior, a well-validated system for the research coding of communications, to code family communications 10 minutes before and 10 minutes after a reflecting team consultation during each initial interview. Family communications coded as "loving and approaching" significantly increased, as communications coded "watching and controlling" and "belittling and blaming" significantly decreased, both changes indicating a shift away from emotional postures of mobilization toward those of tranquility (Griffith et al., 1992).

The reflecting team consultation provides a time in the session where nothing is expected of the patient's family or their therapist, except to listen. Family members, in fact, don't even have to listen to what the reflective team is saying (Roberts, Caesar, Perryclear, & Phillips, 1989). They can allow it to be "background music" and use the time to listen to their own thoughts. Of course, it does not take a team of other therapists to create a space in therapy for listening. A space for reflection can be created through collaborative silence, in a conversation with another family member that includes a plan for the "listener" to be silent and to mull over what is said, or in a conversation with another clinician, nurse, or physician that is structured so that the patient can overhear. Imelda McCarthy and Nollaig Byrne (1988) have likened such dialogical spaces to the imaginary "Fifth Province" of Celtic mythology, where citizens of the Irish four provinces could find, in times of conflict and discord, "a neutral ground where things can detach themselves from all partisan and prejudiced connection" (Hederman & Kearney, 1982, p. 10).

Using the Reflecting Position to Unbind the Body

Creating a reflecting position frequently counters the same social practices that perpetuated the mind-body problems for which treatment was initiated. Gemma Fiumara (1990), in asking why there seems to be so little listening in our society, notes that in daily life there is a felt pressure to negate all that does not fit one's dominant tradition. Whether the dominant tradition is one partner's viewpoint in a marriage, a "family position," or a political or religious agenda in a community, the response by a dominant tradition to dissident voices is typically that of censorship. Power, as Bakhtin (1981) noted, is taking a space in the discourse. These cultural practices give rise to a displacement theory of knowledge, in which the loudest, most aggressive, or most persuasive voice erases all prior knowledge from other voices.

It is difficult to experience alternatives to a dominant perspective when one is addressed directly by that perspective, but one can see its limitations when witnessing it addressing another person. Fiumara (1990, p. 58), although writing as a philosopher, characterized reflecting position techniques in her analysis of listening: "The bewitchment of these authoritative voices appears to persist as long as they address us directly (as when we attend a lecture or read a book) and when the voice speaks to someone else and we perceive the interaction, an inner awakening recreates a critical distance, a philosophical vis or virtus, in the same way as glimpsing how a conjuror performs a trick."

The use of the reflecting position in this sense is in essence a political act whose function is to distribute power among all the different voices in the discourse, dominant and nondominant. The clinician thereby renounces a monopoly that is implicitly conferred by society on the clinician as a professional to dominate exclusively the therapeutic discourse. The gain for the clinician is the melding of perspectives that can bring forth a new reality in which the body of the patient is freed from its binds.

CHAPTER 9

A Complete Therapy

W<small>E CAN AT THIS POINT</small> look at how all the pieces we have thus far discussed fit into the whole of a therapy as it extends from its beginning to its end. These pieces include: (1) creating a conversational domain; (2) identifying unspeakable dilemmas that generate mind-body symptoms; (3) locating binding self-narratives that anchor these dilemmas; and (4) using language skills to escape the influences of binding self-narratives.

We began the story of Mrs. Carson in chapter 2, telling how she had been disabled from work for nearly a decade with seizures that had been shown to be nonepileptic by her neurologists. Shamed and embittered by the new diagnosis, the family, Mr. and Mrs. Carson and their two sons, agreed reluctantly to come for a family therapy consultation. I (JLG) listened to their angry story.

Session One

MR. CARSON: Well, it is just like my wife told you a while ago. She agreed to be taken off the Depakote [an anticonvulsant drug]. She said, "Look, if it is not epileptic seizures, that's fine. I don't care. Just tell me what it is. You know, tell me what you can do about it, what you can do for me!" . . . That's the position, really, of the entire family. We're looking at you. And we are looking at these other professionals—medical people—to give us some answers. And, hell, you are having confusion yourselves.

Can you imagine how confused we might be? . . . We get one doctor over here telling us one thing, and another doctor over there telling us another thing, and another one over here telling us something else.

MRS. CARSON: Well, I had two doctors within just 12 hours tell me totally different things. Dr. Simpson told me Tegretol [another anticonvulsant drug] won't do any good, while Dr. Major told me I had to take it for the rest of my life. I feel like Dr. Simpson doesn't want to have anything to do with me. . . . Total opposites. . . . Dr. Major says: "You need 1,000 mg of Tegretol every day." . . . Dr. Simpson walks in and says: "You don't have epilepsy. There is nothing wrong with you. You don't even need to take any medicine."

MR. CARSON: Right here in this hospital! Two different doctors . . . supposed to be the same type of doctor . . . practitioners of the same medicine . . . to tell her two different things. . . . Buddy, if that don't make you mad as hell, you're not human!

JLG: Uh-huh.

MRS. CARSON: Where does that leave me?

MR. CARSON: Where does that leave the patient? These people get paid too much money for that kind of stuff.

When the session appeared to be deteriorating toward an unsatisfactory end, I finally asked Mr. Carson, "If our positions were switched, and you were here conducting the interview, what would you do?" "I would just try to understand what it must have felt like." I asked, "What did it feel like?" I then sat quietly and listened to their stories of frustration, about enormous medical bills, a wife and mother who stayed ill with seizures, and little to show for the money they had spent. They agreed to return for a second session the next week.

Session Two

Meeting again with all four family members, I asked what things they had noticed from their experiences of living together with the seizures that would suggest why they were getting worse now. This turned out to be a confusing question. They each assumed the seizures were worse, because she was not taking an effective medication. Mr. Carson spoke for the family in stating emphatically, "We can't say, because we don't even know what is physical and what is not. We are not doctors."

I responded in both/and language: "Every neurologist knows that life stress makes epileptic seizures worse. You expect to see a student's seizures at exam time get worse, especially if she starts losing sleep while staying up late studying. And if seizures are not epileptic and are related to psychological things, then of course you expect to see them get worse with stress. You have gone the rounds with the medications, and, in my opinion, that has been unproductive. Are there any things, in your lives, in relationships, anywhere, that your gut tells you might have something to do with the seizures?"

Mr. Carson told how he had recently been hospitalized for cardiac catheterization for an irregular heart beat and recently had started taking antiarrhythmic medications. The family members were apprehensive, about both Mr. Carson's health and the financial threat of his illness, as he provided the sole source of family income. Mrs. Carson felt guilty, believing she needed to work to help the family, but she was unable to do so, because employers either would not hire a person with epilepsy or she would be dismissed when a seizure occurred at work. If the seizures were not epileptic and something else could be done, she wanted to know.

Session Three

I questioned Mrs. Carson closely about exactly what she experienced in her body when her seizures came. She described a tightness in her stomach and tension in her neck and head. If she were to think about these sensations as a readiness for her body to do something, what would that something be? "To run," she said.

If she were to flip back through the pages of her life story, which parts of it most tightly connected with this emotional posture? She then told how she grew up in the explosive atmosphere of a home in which the parents were determined to keep her psychotic older brother with them, rather than in an institution. She recalled her terror in grade school when her brother would sneak up on her while she was sleeping and scream in her ear. She remembered other times when the brother would incorporate her and a sister into his delusions, the three of them boarding furniture against the bedroom doors and standing with knives ready to protect themselves against villains who the psychotic brother believed would soon attack.

Her mother had been chronically ill throughout her childhood, lying in bed for days on end with illnesses that were never well defined. She would often tell the children, "Mother won't be here much longer."

Mrs. Carson's only bright memories were those with her father, who, to her sorrow, was usually away from home traveling as a salesman.

Sessions Four through Seven

I continued meeting every 2 to 3 weeks with Mr. and Mrs. Carson. Their sons could not continue coming because of jobs they were starting. My efforts were devoted to asking questions of authentic curiosity that enabled the important stories of their experience to be fully articulated, particularly those stories that had not been spoken.

We worked to identify which self-narratives from her childhood seemed to be most closely connected with occurrences of her seizures, and which of these tended to be resurrected in the moment-to-moment experiences of her daily life. This inquiry led to practical steps that could limit the intrusion of these old stories into her current life. For example, Mrs. Carson told how her husband was accustomed to loud talking and boisterous arguing, as he grew up with many brothers. But when he and her sons argued loudly, fearful memories from her childhood with her brother flashed before her. On hearing this, Mr. Carson took steps to curtail the arguing or to conduct it outside in the yard. With these measures, Mrs. Carson began to report a modest decrease in the frequency of her seizures.

As she carefully observed the occurrence of her seizures, Mrs. Carson discovered that they did not happen randomly. They were most likely to occur when she was trying her hardest not to have one, especially when visiting in her mother-in-law's home or when applying for a job. These observations might have suggested to some an operant-conditioning paradigm, that her seizures received positive reinforcement, because she, through them, could avoid being with her mother-in-law with whom her relationship was strained, and because she could avoid working. Others might have speculated about unconscious motivations that determined why her seizures occurred at these times. I viewed both such accounts as dormative explanations (Bateson, 1972), in that they put one's critical faculties asleep by explaining everything while providing no effective avenue for action. That is, the reinforcement contingencies with her mother-in-law and work environments would lie outside the control of a clinician, and she had neither the time nor resources for a lengthy therapy devoted to exploring her unconscious mind. As an alternative, viewing her seizures as occurring when she found herself in an unspeakable dilemma could account equally well for her observations, would constitute a much less pathologizing explanation, and would offer far more practical possibilities for designing a therapy.

Session Eight

Most of the time Mrs. Carson could not identify particular emotions by name, although we could talk about the specific physical sensations she felt in her body. "I don't know what I feel," she said repeatedly.

Tonight, however, she returned with a surprise—her discovery and naming of an emotion.

JLG: I always keep connecting it back, you know, to the questions: What would be the kind of environment that would make your seizures worse? What would be the kind of environment that would make them better?

MRS. CARSON: There is one thing—I have developed a sever hatred for my mother. I mean it's very severe. I almost wish Mother would die. Mother torments me. Those are things that really, really bother me. To me, this bothers me more than any of the other relationships we have talked about. It is just eating at me like a cancer. I hate my mother. I do . . . I just hate her. And I don't really feel bad about hating her. But I don't feel that it is good for anyone to hate.*

JLG: Is this something that is changing as we have spent time talking about things here?

MRS. CARSON: The feelings of hate have grown deeper and deeper.

JLG: And you hate having those kinds of thoughts?

MRS. CARSON: No, I really don't. But I hate the kind of person I am turning into.

JLG: How are you finding the thoughts to be shaping who you are?

MRS. CARSON: For one thing, I haven't been having nearly as many seizures.

JLG: How do you understand that?

MRS. CARSON: I don't know. I'm not having nearly as many seizures, but I know I'm being ugly.

MR. CARSON: I personally think what is happening to her—I've learned a lot from these sessions—is that it is like when we were talking about her separating her emotions . . . how did we describe that?

MRS. CARSON: I would detach myself.

MR. CARSON: Detaching herself from her body . . . her feelings from her body. I think she is beginning to learn how not to do that. That is what I think—I am not a professional.

JLG: [To Mrs. Carson] How does that theory sound to you?

MRS. CARSON: I think that is what it really is.

JLG: So is it like the anger—the word you used was "hatred"—the hatred you are feeling is not a new emotion? Is it like it is just now entering your body?

MRS. CARSON: I hate my mother. I think I have always hated her, but I have masked it.

JLG: Is that better for it to be inside your body, rather than to be detached from your body?

---

*There is a complexity of meaning for Mrs. Carson's statements that is not evident from the literal transcript. As she said on a number of occasions, she continued to love her mother and to be committed to her, even as she stated, "I hate my mother." "Hate" was, in a sense, an addition to many mixed feelings she had toward her mother, and it was part of their story together that had not been acknowledged.

MRS. CARSON: Oh, I think it's better for it to be inside my body. I don't know from a Christian standpoint if that is a Christian way to feel. I have a problem with that. Because I know that, according to the Bible, it is not right to hate people.

JLG: If your body could speak, what would it say about the presence of the hatred?

MRS. CARSON: Hey, this feels good. . . . You know, for once in my life my body feels good.

JLG: When you say "feel good," what are you actually feeling in your body?

MRS. CARSON: I feel *feeling*. I feel the feeling *hate*.

JLG: Uh-huh.

MRS. CARSON: You see, I used not to feel anything—except that I would be frightened by whatever it was that maybe I did feel. But I'm not scared of it anymore. I feel more relaxed.

JLG: More relaxed. With the feeling inhabiting your body, rather than the feeling being on the outside?

MRS. CARSON: Yes.

JLG: I was wondering whether it was that kind of relaxation that you were connecting to the seizures being less frequent, or were you relating it to something else?

MRS. CARSON: Possibly. I know that with the seizures being less frequent, my mind doesn't feel like it is in a turmoil a lot.

JLG: Your mind and your body are relaxing together?

MRS. CARSON: It is like I'm not fighting my mind. My body used to say, "Missy, don't feel that way." I would have the feelings in my mind, and I would try to suppress them and shut them down. . . . It makes me nervous to sit here and to tell you that I hate my mother, because I know it is not a Christian thing to do, and I have strong Christian convictions. . . . But I cannot deny that I hate her. I mean, I cannot deny those feelings.

JLG: Where do you place this acknowledgment of your feelings in a Christian context? I mean, do you see it as more Christian or less Christian to acknowledge your feelings?

MRS. CARSON: Well, I feel like if you hate someone, you really cannot have a relationship with God, unless you go to God with that problem. And it is hard to go to God with hate in your heart.

JLG: I guess I was thinking . . . if God were looking down, do you think he would prefer that you speak, that you acknowledge or confess the feelings, or that you detach from them?

MRS. CARSON: Knowing God the way I know him, he would rather I be truthful with him and tell him, "You know, God, I hate my mother. I don't know how to deal with this. It may not be pleasing to you. But I do hate her."

JLG: So is this like a step toward God?

MRS. CARSON: Yes, in a way it is. In a way it is.

JLG: You know, as I listen, I think back to our first meeting and the question of the seizures. What is the path toward healing? What is the path away from healing? In thinking about your finding hatred flowing into and inhabiting your body, I ask myself the question: Is the hatred on the side of healing, or is it on the side away from healing?

MRS. CARSON: I hope it is on the side of healing.

JLG: This might be a good time to get some thoughts from our colleagues. They have had a chance to listen to and reflect on what we have been talking about. We can get some of their thoughts, then we can come back and talk some more.

[The reflecting team members—Melissa (MEG), Ian Law, Vanessa Law, and Lynn Joseph—and the family members and JLG switch places, the reflecting team now sitting in the therapy room and the family with JLG now watching from the observation room.]

MEG: As Mrs. Carson described the sense of release and freedom she felt when she acknowledged her true feelings of hatred for her mother and her dilemma that this could grow and eat at her like a cancer, I was really curious to know what all of the voices were inside of her, and among those what the voice of God might be. She said that there was a still, small voice that said, "If you aren't good to your mother, you don't love the Lord Jesus." I started to wonder about all the meanings of "being good to your mother." She has been doing the one of fulfilling her obligations, of being good to her mother in that way. But I started to wonder if "being good to your mother" could ever be expanded to mean "being honest with your mother." What would "being good to your mother" mean if she were looking at it from the standpoint of herself as a mother? What does she want from her own children? What does it mean to be good to your mother in the deepest sense, even if your mother can't receive the goodness immediately?

VANESSA: I hear that this family holds dear the values of honesty and care toward a mother and her children. These values they hold so dear are values of the Christian faith. Surely, they are the values her mother taught her. Maybe, living true to those values is a way "to be good to your mother."

IAN: I've heard someone say that you have to embrace something before you can let it go. Maybe only now can she begin to let it go. She talked about loosening the ball and chain around her neck. Maybe, she can begin to loosen the hatred.

LYNN: I like what you said, Ian, about holding on to this, so that she can let it go. I see this as a part of the process. There was a lot of conversation about feeling more whole in mind and body. Hatred has always had a connotation of being a nasty word. But I am just wondering if it can't be something that at this point isn't working toward wholeness and is just part of the process that is not always going to be part of her mind and part of her body. I just got a sense of Mrs. Carson's disempowering these seizures, and she did it by empowering herself. She's getting her own picture clearly, not living by her mother's picture.

[After a few related comments, the team members end by acknowledging how supportive Mr. Carson had been of his wife, despite his difficult and demoralizing work situation. The reflecting team again switch places with the family and me to return to their respective rooms.]

JLG: Well, they had a number of comments. I wondered whether there were any things that resonated with your experience? . . . Were there any things that struck a chord?

MR. CARSON: Sometimes, I feel like I'm punching in the dark. To sit here and have them say the things about me they did—it makes me feel I'm on the right track.

MRS. CARSON: When I went into that room to listen to them talk, I was so cold. My hands were icy, but as they began to speak, my whole body began to warm up, and I relaxed. It was very soothing. It was almost tranquilizing.

JLG: Which comments were the most soothing . . . the most tranquilizing?

MRS. CARSON: Every comment made me feel a little better about myself, that I am not a bad person—just because I feel the feeling of hatred and I acknowledge it. I feel like it is a starting point. I don't know where it will go, but I know it will go, and this is the start.

JLG: The speed has really been astounding so far, faster than I ever would have guessed. I'm not sure I really understand it.

There were multiple unspeakable dilemmas in Mrs. Carson's life, more than can be contained in a summary account of a therapy. The dilemma discussed here was a particularly difficult one and serves as a model for how the others were addressed: Mrs. Carson's relationship with her personal God was a vital relationship on which she had relied through many times of pain and struggle. She believed that a person cannot stand in the presence of God with hatred in her heart for another person. Yet, her emotional posture, consistent with the self-narratives within which she lived, was that of hatred. There was no other person with whom this dilemma could be talked about. If feelings are a person's self-report as to the body's emotion, then her solution to the dilemma had been to disregard the report, that is, "to feel nothing."

As we created a language and a relationship, conversation about the dilemma became possible. Questions could then be asked that invited a reauthoring of the story, from that of "I betray God by hating" to "I show my trust of God by acknowledging the hatred I feel." With this reauthoring, her dilemma remained, but it no longer would be held in silence.

In the interview there are illustrations of a variety of reflective questions. The question, "If God were looking down, do you think he would prefer...," served a dual role. It invited Mrs. Carson to move to an alternative epistemological position, that of the external observer, that reliably would bring a different perspective to her situation. It also initiated a sequence of questions that facilitated the restoration of intimacy in her relationship with her God. This intrapersonal relationship had been a powerful source of soothing and comfort in the past and could become such again in the future.

The question, "If your body could speak, what would it say...," created a dialogical space in the relationship for her body. When the body has a voice in a conversation, it seldom must communicate by pantomime through somatic symptoms.

Sessions Nine through Sixteen

The pace of change in Mrs. Carson's life and that of her family speeded up. Within her story, using her language, with my always consulting to her own path of discovery, we came up with a number of actions that she and the family could take. Most of these were simple and commonsense and required no expert knowledge for their conceptualization. Her siblings had turned to her over the years to look after her mother. Her mother, continuing to live with the psychotic son was, as she had been during childhood, chronically ill with many different somatoform symptoms, always telling her children that she would be dying soon. Mrs. Carson decided that she could not be both well from her seizures and also in regular contact with her mother. She informed her siblings that they would need to look after the mother, and she obtained an unlisted telephone number, so that she could not be called unless she initiated the call.

She began confronting some of her in-laws, which led to a crisis in her husband's family. She insisted that her adult sons accept greater responsibility for their life decisions and the consequences of those decisions. She successfully interviewed for a job as a secretary.

Her seizures had greatly diminished, although some did still occur. A particular difficulty arose when she was in a situation that she knew to be risky for a seizure, but from which she did not have the option of leaving. For example, her boss, Norman, would give her several pieces of work with immediate deadlines. But then he would drop by her desk to chat. She knew that he would be furious if the work were not to be completed on time. But he was a domineering man, and she did not feel that she could decline to talk with him when he stopped by. Sitting worried and frustrated, yet pretending to be friendly and relaxed while talking to Norman, triggered a seizure more than once and eventually led to her leaving her job.

Session Seventeen

JLG: What do you do exactly at the moment that you are starting to sense that a spell is coming on? What is your signal?

MRS. CARSON: Well, I'll start feeling like, you know, that things are kind of getting fuzzy in my head, and I'll say, "Okay, Missy, calm down. You're upset." What kind of upset? Am I angry? Am I mad? Am I sad? Am I scared? And it is like my brain starts slowing down, and I start thinking about, "What am I?" at that moment. And then, if I realize that I am scared, I'll think, "Well, sit down and calm down. What are you scared about? What are you afraid of?"

JLG: Let me ask you something. When you are talking to yourself in that way: "Sit down. Calm down. What are you afraid of?" . . . Whose voice in your life does that remind you of?

MRS. CARSON: [Pause] My father's.

JLG: Are you kind of talking to yourself as your father would? That is what I was wondering.

MRS. CARSON: Yeah.

JLG: So your father still lives on within you in a way?

MRS. CARSON: Yes, he does. . . . I dreamed of him very, very much right after he died. . . . And I would get very, very upset. I would have these dreams of my father, and he would always take me by the hand, and he would say, "It is all going to be okay, sweetheart. It is all going to be okay. Now, there is nothing to be afraid of. You're going to be fine." He was a very reassuring person. He was a very kind person. He was a very good listener . . . I don't know. It was that voice. I hadn't thought about it until you asked me that. I guess it is my father's.

JLG: Let me ask you this question: This being presented to you in a dream, as a memory that you have . . . you can keep it . . . you can access it . . . would that be something that you can actively and deliberately use when you find yourself going into one of these spells?

MRS. CARSON: Oh, yes. The dreams were so real that I would wake up, and I honestly felt as if I could smell my father's aftershave on my hand. And I know that is stupid and I couldn't, but the dream was just that real to me. And I can still—that's been 9 years since he died—the grass . . . walking by the bird bath . . . talking to me in his voice.

JLG: You know, whenever you have been in a situation like at your desk as a secretary with your boss, Norman . . . in the midst of that situation . . . have you ever called up your father's presence?

MRS. CARSON: No. I usually kind of get dizzy or feel like I'm going to have a spell.

JLG: Whether that be by speaking to yourself or to imagine walking—see the sights ... the bird bath ... smell his aftershave—really call up his presence in the midst of the situation you can't get out of.

MRS. CARSON: Did I do it when I was working there? No, I didn't.

JLG: Because, you know, we started this conversation with your asking me, "But what can I do?"

MRS. CARSON: So that would be one thing maybe I could do? Something to try out?

JLG: Yeah, something to try out. Let's look at the outcome of it and see how it works.

Session Eighteen

JLG: When you were away from here, outside the room, working on this, which parts of your own work do you think contributed most to the changes?

MRS. CARSON: Which parts of my own work?

JLG: Yes. Of the things that you really worked on ... and practiced ... and struggled with when at home.

MRS. CARSON: It was like I could hear your voice over and over and over again: "If your body could speak, what would it say?" Because, when you first said that to me, I said, "Yeah, I know he is a psychiatrist, but this is really squirrely." But, you know, for some reason that sunk into my head, and that one phrase—I would bring that up, "Now, Missy, if your body could speak, what would it say?" ... And it got to where it just came all the time, "If your body could speak, what would it say?" ... And my body would just start saying things.

JLG: Were there ever any other questions I ever asked that seemed to be particularly helpful?

MRS. CARSON: Questions? ... Well, that one was the most difficult. You asked me lots of questions, but that was the only one that seemed to come out from left field ... and that was the only one that I seemed to work with the most. ... That's strange! ... I thought, "Why in the world is he asking me this?"

MR. CARSON: Well, I think, for me, in relation to her, "What was going on? What was the situation at the time that she would feel the seizure coming on?"

MRS. CARSON: I know another question, too, that was a very vital one: "Is it the feeling you are feeling, or is it you trying to stop the feeling?" And it was just like your voice was a recording in my brain. And it was just like daily I could hear you going over and over asking me those questions. And it was true. It really wasn't the feeling. It was me trying to shut it down. Because when I tried to shut the feeling down a couple of times, I remember, I hit the floor.

JLG: Okay. By the way, how have things been? I told you I would ask you specifically what you have noticed about situations that bring on the spells. We talked about that some last time.

MRS. CARSON: Well, I remember what you told me. I have been trying really hard when I feel like I might be going to have a spell, with feelings like anger, or fear, sometimes just loneliness, I try to really work through those feelings. . . . And I worked really hard to bring back that image of the dream I had of my father. . . . And, fortunately, I think I'm having a great deal of success. It's really amazing. It's just like I can just—a lady came over to my house, and she is into this New Age movement. She was discussing some things with me, and I felt a little hostility. I felt kind of angry, because I told her I really didn't want to discuss that, and she wouldn't stop. I felt myself getting really, really angry. When she left, I knew that I was angry. And then I thought, "It is okay to be angry, but you need to calm down." I pulled the memory back up—the dream, the grass, the bird bath, the whole thing—and that feeling began to diminish.

JLG: I still wonder about—and I guess I wish you would just notice care-fully—do you ever have spells when you are truly in that state of deep relaxation? Or are those the right words? What words would you use to describe it?

MRS. CARSON: It is just a real warm feeling that fills my body . . . a very calm-ing feeling.

JLG: I wish you would notice whether you ever have a seizure when you are in that warm, calming feeling, or whether they come exclusively out of some of those torn positions where you feel pulled in two ways, between being angry and trying not to show anger. [Pause] You know, this dream of your father is like a piece of gold ore that has been there for a long time that you reached down and picked up. It has been there . . . for years. You know, I wonder whether there are any other things lying around that you could make use of—very good, or very desirable, mem-ories of times in your life that you really can take yourself back to, and go into . . . by imagining being at that place . . . what the sounds were . . . what the sights were . . . even smells in the air, if there were any.

MRS. CARSON: I wonder what made me dream that dream after my father's death?

JLG: I won't try to explain it. I mean, I see things like that happen. What I said last time is that I see it as a gift. Something given to you that you needed to learn how to use. Something that he left for you.

Many unspeakable dilemmas are real-life dilemmas, in the sense that they do not disappear by viewing them from a different perspective. Usually, such dilemmas have to do with power inequities in relationships, such as Mrs. Carson's relationship with her boss, in which the person in power is threatened or angered by differences or dissidence or is exploitive of the power. Yet, as Mrs. Carson discovered, there are domains of relationships that exist within a person where one can turn for the caring, soothing, and protection that can enable one's body to remain within emotional postures of tranquility despite a hostile outside world.

Mrs. Carson's story took a final ironic turn. After limiting all contact with her mother for 6 months, she returned to say that she did not want to bear any longer the complete severing of contact, even at the price of having more seizures. As we examined all the changes in her life, we agreed that she was in fact at a very different, stronger place now. I expressed confidence that we could deal with whatever consequences there might be.

She made a surprise visit to her mother, only to find that her mother was a transformed person. Rather than obsessing over her somatoform complaints, her mother was more interested in conversing about all the events happening in the world. The mother listened to her daughter, opening the way for conversations that they had never before had about their life together and how her mother had never really recovered from the death of her husband years before.

A few months after Mrs. Carson had broken contact, an old psychiatrist whom she occasionally visited had died. One of Mrs. Carson's siblings took the mother to a young psychiatrist who specialized in geriatric psychiatry. He prescribed Zoloft, an antidepressant. Within a few days, the mother blossomed, showing an interest in living that by their memories she had never before shown. Her mother told Mrs. Carson that she had been depressed for 20 years and now realized the bad effect it had on her family. Since then, Mrs. Carson and her mother have spent many good times together on visits.

CHAPTER 10

Ethological Pharmacology

MRS. YOUNG, a recovered alcoholic, confessed that she had been lax in following her recovery program during the past year. For 7 years of sobriety, she had zealously attended her Alcoholics Anonymous (AA) meetings, had repeatedly taken her moral inventory, and had worked daily to hold on to the sense of powerlessness over alcohol on which a 12-step recovery program is built. These had been years of struggle, however, in which she stoically focused on enduring one day until the next. Then, she discovered Prozac. Suddenly the anxiety and depression that fed her hunger for alcohol evaporated. The struggle for sobriety that had been so difficult for so long now seemed effortless. With relief and delight, she let go of her pharisaical adherence to the 12-step philosophy. Her AA meeting attendance went from three times a week to once monthly. Abstinence came easily for her.

But now she felt both guilty and resentful. Would she be punished by her lapses? Was she foolhardy in challenging fate by relaxing her recovery program? Or had she been duped—had the problem all along been a "chemical imbalance" that simply needed the right medication, like other diseases needed their specific medications for a cure? Lacking a general theory that explains how change through language and change through pharmacology both occur, clinicians and patients alike often feel confused. Will pharmacology replace the "talking therapies" when we finally understand which drug should be used to treat which psychiatric disorder? Do medications simply bury problems, rather than deal with them as do the talking therapies? Do pharmacological therapies and language-based therapies compete with one another, counteract one another, or potentiate each other's effectiveness?

The Misdirection of Pharmacological Therapy in American Psychiatry

Much of the confusion and uncertainty about how to use pharmacological therapies and conversational therapies is fostered by ideologies that became dominant in psychiatry during the last half-century.

Psychopharmacology is a name adopted by the subdiscipline within psychiatry that mainly relies on medications for treating patients. Once a minor segment of the field, psychopharmacology now dominates American psychiatry, both in academic research and training centers and in clinical practice. Most psychopharmacologists view the mind and the brain as synonomous, – and, like neurologists and neurosurgeons, consider themselves to be physicians of the brain. Acknowledging the emerging dominance of psychopharmacology within psychiatry, Congress declared the 1990s to be the "Decade of the Brain."

It is widely assumed that the rapid growth of psychopharmacology was propelled by dramatic breakthroughs in finding new medications for symptoms, such as anxiety, psychosis, and depression, that had responded poorly to the traditional psychotherapies. This is true to a surprisingly limited extent. Nearly all classes of medications used by psychopharmacologists in the 1990s had been synthesized during the 1950s. A cover-story article in *Time* magazine in 1992 (Wallis & Willwerth, 1992), for example, featured the drug clozapine as the exemplar for the rapid advances in drug treatments of schizophrenia, even though clozapine was synthesized in 1960 and was available in countries other than the United States years ago (Safferman, Lieberman, Kane, Szymanski, & Kinon, 1991). In fact, almost all of the drugs discussed in the *Time* magazine article were available for clinical use, at least in prototype, by 1960 (Wallis & Willwerth, 1992; Elmer-Dewitt, 1992; Hollister & Csernansky, 1990).

Moreover, truly new drug classes, such as Prozac and other serotonin-reuptake inhibitors, have added little increased treatment efficacy compared to the drugs that were available three decades ago, although they usually have fewer side effects. This statement may seem startling and in need of justification given the popular enthusiasm for recent books, such as Peter Kramer's (1993) *Listening to Prozac,* that document transformed lives after medications for persons disabled by phobias, depression, or compulsive behaviors. Part of this incongruity can be explained by the lack of public awareness for what can be accomplished with psychiatric medications that have been with us since the 1950s. The rest of the explanation is that psychiatrists since 1980 have been discovering that the old drugs can perform new tricks. Anafranil and Clozaril, both 1950s vintage drugs, were not marketed for treatment of obsessive-compulsive symptoms and treatment-resistant schizophrenia until the 1990s. Then, too, the lack of side effects of a new generation of antidepressants, such as Prozac, Paxil, Zoloft, and Wellbutrin, has meant that persons unwilling or unable to tolerate the older drugs could take the new ones with little bother. There is no strong evidence that Prozac works differently or is any more potent than Anafranil or fluvoxamine (another old antidepressant still not marketed in the U.S.) for any of the symptoms to which it has been applied. But its absence of side effects has meant that Americans would take it by the millions.

This increasing recognition and acceptability of drug treatments has obscured a lack of truly new ideas in the field since the 1950s and 1960s. Drug treatment in psychiatry is better today, but the difference is more like comparing the internal combustion engines of the 1950s to today's engines with better fuel efficiencies and less pollution, rather than to a truly new engine. As new drugs are developed that selectively block or potentiate sub-types of noradrenergic, serotonergic, and dopaminergic receptors in the brain, the same vein may be mined a bit longer. But one wonders whether the end is in sight where, without greater innovation, drug treatment in psychiatry will stall in its progress. Breakthroughs in new drugs alone could not have provided the impetus for the explosive growth of drug treatments witnessed in psychiatry.

If advances in developing new drugs seem to have played only a secondary role in fueling the rapid expansion of psychopharmacology as a professional discipline, then changes in how psychiatric problems were diagnosed played a primary role. These changes resulted in a psychiatric diagnostic system that fit well the medication treatment of psychiatric symptoms but fit poorly the treatment of symptoms by other means. The DSM-III diagnostic system, sometimes now called the "Bible of psychiatry" (Chase, 1993), was an effort to create for psychiatry diagnoses that resembled the physiology-based diagnoses that characterized diagnosis and treatment in other medical specialties, such as cardiology or gastroenterology, where medications and surgery are the therapies.

There were a number of reasons why psychiatrists in the 1970s and 1980s wanted to resemble more closely their medical colleagues in their clinical practices. The maturing of psychology, social work, psychiatric nursing, and licensed professional counseling as mental health disciplines added huge numbers of professionals conducting psychotherapy to the mental health care marketplace. Many of these nonphysician psychotherapists were trained in psychotherapies that were as effective, but briefer and less expensive, than the psychoanalytic therapies to which psychiatry was wedded. Many psychiatrists felt they could not compete with nonphysician mental health providers. Psychiatrists' incomes were near the bottom among the various medical specialties. Proposals for national health care reform raised the possibility that medical treatments, yet not psychotherapy, would be funded in the future health care systems. Morale in psychiatry fell lower and lower, and its ranks thinned as medical school graduates abandoned psychiatry for other careers. For these and other reasons, psychiatry sought vigorously to realign itself with its fellow medical disciplines, rather than the non-physician mental health disciplines. But the way psychiatric problems were diagnosed stood in the way. Because psychiatric symptoms were as likely to arise from social, family, economic, and political problems as from physiological problems, the complexity of psychiatric diagnoses dispelled any vague similarity to precise, narrowly defined medical diagnoses, such as appendicitis, pneumonia, or leukemia.

In the 1960s and 1970s, psychiatric academicians, largely organized around the Washington University School of Medicine, published a series of research papers that appeared to eliminate the complexity that troubled psychiatric nosology (Goodwin & Guze, 1984). These academicians made an a priori assumption that the individual patient was the unit of psychopathology (American Psychiatric Association, 1987). This assumption hid from view relationships between psychiatric symptoms expressed by an individual patient and a multitude of events occurring in his or her family, social community, religious community, political system, or economic system. Many nonphysician mental health professionals cried, "Foul play!," but the DSM-III diagnostic system was accepted by governmental agencies and insurance companies, thereby ensuring its dominance. By 1990, 10% to 20% of all prescriptions in America were written to affect mental processes (Baldessarini, 1990). Fitted with a diagnostic system that magnified physiological contributions to psychiatric symptoms, while minimizing social contributions, psychopharmacology became a growth industry both for pharmaceutical corporations and for psychiatry as a professional guild.

However successful DSM-III has been as a political and economic document, its lack of relevance for nonpharmacological treatments has limited the ability of clinicians to treat patients by means other than medications. This shackling has perhaps been most pronounced for the mind-body problems that have been the focus of this book—somatoform symptoms for which pharmacological treatments have little to offer. But throughout the mental health disciplines, this nosology has led to ways of thinking about pharmacological treatments that actually curtailed their potential efficacy in the hands of psychiatrists and often rendered them unusable for nonphysician mental health providers.

Ethological Pharmacology, Not Psychopharmacology

Ethology is the scientific study of animal behavior in the interest of understanding the formation of human character. Ethologists describe and classify the different repertoires of behaviors that animals employ in creating their

social worlds of mating, establishing dominance, cooperating, claiming territory, parenting, and other activities. The performance of these social interactions is regulated by the same brain systems that most of our psychiatric
medications influence. Ethological pharmacology is the planned effort to
bias the occurrence of particular classes of social behavior, such as increasing
assertiveness or diminishing irritability, by resetting these brain systems
with medications. A primary agenda is to use medications in ways that create new possibilities for conversation and relationships.

During and after her therapy for nonepileptic seizures, Mrs. Carson, as
seen in chapter 9, continued to take diazepam (Valium), a benzodiazepine
medication, on a daily basis, because she felt her control over her seizures to
be more secure. Years earlier, she had discovered its beneficial effects herself
when her family physician had prescribed it. The drug did not stop her
seizures, but she had noticeably fewer seizures when taking it. In her therapy with me (JLG), I did not try to stop it but, rather, encouraged her to continue taking it.

Diazepam is a medication that diminishes the alarm response of the body
to threatening circumstances. In taking the diazepam, Ms. Carson felt less
pressured to camouflage her body's expression, while we worked in the
therapy to find paths out of her dilemmas. Our physiology-based and
language-based interventions worked in synchrony toward a common end
of reducing the number of seizures.

How to join physiology-based and language-based therapies to solve clinical problems is clearer if we revisit two ideas already discussed:

1.) Language is a complex form of gesturing, a way of touching the body
    from a distance. Language can reconfigure the physiological state of the
    body, and vice versa.
2.) Emotion is a bodily disposition for action or expression toward the
    other, and as such is always an interpersonal phenomenon.

Language events and physiological events constantly select and constrain
one another via the body's emotion. This dual description of emotional postures provides a conceptual framework for the practice of ethological pharmacology. In chapters 3 and 4 we discussed how to use language to structure physiology. Ethological pharmacology is organized around the other
side of the relationship, using physiology to structure language.

An examination of the function in the natural world of brain systems
through which effects of psychiatric drugs are mediated suggests how best
to understand the actions of the drugs. Psychiatric medications alter the
activity of one or more brain systems that provide some type of "feed-
forward biasing" of sensibility in a relational world. All the so-called
antipsychotic, antianxiety, antidepressant, antibulimic, antiobsessional
drugs act in the body to influence how these systems prepare brain informa-

tion processing for an anticipated future. Like a fighter raising an arm to block an expected punch, they reset the sensitivities of sensory systems, such as sight and hearing, to detect relevant events and to speed transmission of their neuronal signals through brain pathways. When working well, these systems offer a person a competitive advantage by preparing for adversity before it arrives.

These brain systems have been named according to which chemical messenger, or neurotransmitter, is the main conveyer of signals from one brain cell, or neuron, to the next. These include the norepinephrine (noradrenergic), serotonin (serotonergic), dopamine (dopaminergic), acetylcholine (cholinergic), gammahydroxybutyric acid (GABA), and histamine (histaminic) systems. Brain systems targeted by current psychiatric medications are only a half-dozen or so among possibly thousands of systems within the brain. They are unique in that they do not convey sensation into the brain or command the body to move. Rather, they regulate "state functions," meaning that they determine which kinds of perception and information processing are given priority.

Except for the GABA system, cell bodies for these brain systems are located deeply and compactly in the core of the nervous system, extending from the brainstem to the base of the cerebral hemispheres. From this central location, their nerve fibers extend diffusely, reaching far-flung regions of the brain and spinal cord. As a group, they appear to influence how large regions, or even the entire brain, processes its information, even though their own organizational sophistication does not make them capable of transmitting complex information with precision. Their function is one of modulating behavioral states, rather than conveying information with a high degree of fidelity to and from the world outside the person.

As an example, the norepinephrine system is better understood than the others and illustrates well how this regulation of behavioral states works. The nerve cells that constitute the noradrenergic system lie deep in the brainstem, mostly in a tiny nucleus called the locus coeruleus. There they number only 20,000 out of possibly a trillion nerve cells in the brain (Jacobs, 1986; Kandel, 1985). Yet, these few neurons give off long fibers that branch again and again and again, forming a dense network of fibers that eventually reach every area of the cerebral cortex, as well as many other regions of the nervous system, such as the limbic system, cerebellum, and much of the spinal cord. The noradrenergic system is a phylogenetically ancient system, meaning that its structure in the brain of a rat looks much like that in a dog or a monkey or a human (Nieuwenhuys, 1985). This suggests that the noradrenergic system plays a fundamental, but simple, role in the overall functioning of the brain. We may liken it to the light switch in a room that plays a crucially important function in the usability of the room, but whose design has changed little over the years, although the designs of other electrical equipment in the room, such as tape recorders, stereos, computers, and tele-visions, have become progressively more complex and sophisticated over the years.

The noradrenergic system appears to be an alarm system that signals the presence of either novelty or threat in the surrounding world (Clark, Geffan, & Geffan, 1987; Jacobs, 1986). When it discharges, it shifts the orientation of information-processing systems throughout the brain to focus on scanning the person's life-world for a potential threat, and it initiates a behavioral readiness to run or to fight. When the locus coeruleus discharges within the brain, the discharge is accompanied by a simultaneous discharge of the sym-pathetic nervous system elsewhere that readies the rest of the body, by speeding the heart, raising blood pressure, shunting blood away from the internal organs to the arms and legs, and dumping glucose, for fuel, into the bloodstream from its stores in the liver (Jacobs, 1987).

Contrasted with its actions during a state of high activation, the noradren-ergic system grows relatively quiescent when an animal (or human) shows consummatory and grooming behaviors—eating and drinking, grooming self or other, or resting. It falls completely silent during the intensely inwardly directed, creative state of dreaming that occurs during rapid eye movement sleep (Jacobs, 1986).

Judging from these observations, we can surmise that physiological states associated with a strong readiness to respond to environmental threat, evi-denced by high activation of the noradrenergic system, select a domain of psychological states within which reflective listening and the generation of new meaning are unlikely to occur. Conversely, a state of low activation of the noradrenergic system, as in trance induction when the soft, rhythmic words of the hypnotist lull the noradrenergic system into an idling mode, select a domain of psychological states favorable for reflective listening and generation of new meaning.

Similar or complementary descriptions can be made about the choliner-gic, serotonergic, dopaminergic, and histaminic systems. Each of these sys-tems appears to operate by a feed-forward mechanism that biases either (1) which sensed events in the life-world receive preferential access to the ner-vous system; (2) which kind of information receives preferential attention during information processing; or (3) which repertoires of behaviors are made available from which to select one's actions.

When a person presents a problem, such as recurrent panic attacks, it has been shown that his or her noradrenergic system is set at a very high level of sensitivity, establishing a brain readiness for noticing and rapidly respond-ing to life-world events that could be potential threats (Charney et al., 1990). Because many life events are intrinsically ambiguous in their meaning, this early-warning system is constantly setting off false alarms for someone with panic attacks, like a burglar alarm that sounds every time a squirrel walks across the roof. With some persons, this low threshold for alarm appears to be a learned behavior, and with others it appears to result from an inborn instability in either the noradrenergic or serotonergic systems. In any case, the medications effective in stopping panic symptoms, such as alprazolam, imipramine, fluoxetine, and phenelzine, are all shown to turn down, directly or indirectly, the level of activation of the noradrenergic system (Charney et al., 1990).

Changing Physiology to Create New Possibilities for Conversation

Anyone who has attempted to work in therapy with a person who is debilitated by ongoing panic attacks knows how little room there is for therapeutic dialogue. Such a patient often is wholly preoccupied with an idea that his or her palpitating heart, sweaty palms, tremor, and feeling of dread all signal the onset of a dire illness. The patient can focus only on these bodily symptoms, a search for medical treatment to stop them, and avoidance of situations, such as shopping malls, elevators, and churches, that in strange ways seem to trigger them. Not surprisingly, when medications raise the threshold for brain mechanisms for triggering panic behavior, new possibilities appear for open and reflective conversation.

Melanie Hinds, for example, was referred by her psychotherapist for a psychiatric evaluation. The psychotherapist felt strongly that Melanie's bodily symptoms were manifestations of anxiety, but she could not convince Melanie to examine problems that the psychotherapist felt accounted for her anxiety.

Arriving at the session with her mother, Melanie, frightened and agitated, asked for a medical evaluation for her racing heart, tingling hands, and shortness of breath. From their reading in the medical literature, both she and her mother were firmly convinced that she had reactive hypoglycemia and wanted a full medical evaluation. They were both upset that Melanie had been referred to the psychotherapist by her family physician, without being told that the psychotherapist was not a physician. They were frustrated with the family physician, because he had made the referral, rather than pursuing medical diagnostic tests, and they wanted me (JLG) to order the tests. After hearing their full story and myself doubtful that her symptoms could be related to hypoglycemia, I suggested a trial of Xanax first to rule out the possibility that her somatic symptoms were related to panic attacks. Reluctantly, she and her mother agreed that she would take the medication for 4 days, if I would agree to see her back then to order tests for hypoglycemia if she were still symptomatic.

By the next visit, Melanie's somatic symptoms had ceased, and she returned without her mother. Our conversation then moved easily into talk about problems with her boss on a job she hated and her uncertainty about marriage to a man she had been dating, but who, she felt, neglected her emotional needs. She subsequently returned to the psychotherapist who had referred her and worked with her productively in therapy on these issues.

When initially referred, Melanie was so focused on the possible threat to the integrity of her body that neither the psychotherapist nor I could find an opening to begin a dialogue in which she could tell about life experiences that extended beyond her immediate bodily sensations. Indeed, she and her mother agreed to the Xanax trial only because it could be considered a "medical" treatment, and because I agreed to pursue the medical concerns they had if it had not worked. Upon returning, however, she was no longer in emotional postures of mobilization that fixed her gaze on her body so much that she could not see the expanse of her own life story.

We can best think about the action of the Xanax as turning down the sensitivity of Melanie's brain systems for monitoring threat, including both noradrenergic and GABA systems, much as one would turn down a rheostat to dim lights that are shining too bright. This shift to emotional postures of tranquility made possible the selection of psychological states more conducive to conversation and reflective listening. The resetting of her brain systems for monitoring threat did not prescribe that reflective listening would occur for Melanie, nor could an understanding of her reflective listening be reduced to an understanding of the physiology of these brain systems. Their level of sensitivity did, however, strongly condition whether reflective listening would be permitted to occur. Changing physiology can create new possibilities for change through language.

Detailed study of physiological mechanisms in the brain can be a fruitful way to inspire the synthesis of new drugs. However, an understanding of these physiological mechanisms can no more shed light on their potential meaning in the life-worlds of patients and families than would a schematic diagram of the electronic circuitry of a compact disk player handed to an alien from Mars enable the alien to understand the possibilities it could bring for experiencing Mozart. We can only gain this understanding of brain systems by looking directly at the social worlds people live within. Biological psychiatrists, with rare exceptions, have been too preoccupied with the mechanics of the brain systems to think deeply about these systems' social significance or that of the medications they prescribe.

We propose that clinicians discontinue the practice of psychopharmacology—as "drug treatment of the mind"—in describing and understanding the role of pharmacological treatment in their clinical settings. Ethological pharmacology, by pointing to possibilites and contraints that can be imposed on a social world by pharmacological treatments, offers a way of thinking about medications that is more useful for clinicians who plan a more comprehensive and complex therapy than simply prescribing a pill. A pharmacoethologist thinks about how medications can create the physiological space for the appearance of new language and new meaning that will be transformative and therapeutic for the patient and his or her social relationships.

Patients and Family Members as Partners in Clinical Decision Making

An ethological approach to pharmacology creates new possibilities for partnership between a clinician and a patient that would not exist for a psychopharmacologist treating a presumed psychiatric illness that resides in the patient's body. The clinical aim of ethological pharmacology is not to treat a patient's disease or disorder but, by understanding sociophysiological relationships, to include medications as one of the ways to assist in opening new possibilities for conversation and social relationships.

The first task of pharmacoethological treatment is to build a language together, a conversational domain, within which the clinician and patient can talk together about physiology and medications. What does taking a medication mean to a patient and the patient's family? Are there stories from the past, good or bad, about experiences with medications in treating similar symptoms? Are there family stories about medication treatment for symptoms of emotion, thought, and behavior? What metaphors constitute the patient's language in talking about medications? An understanding of medication and its actions in the body is best elaborated within a patient's language whenever possible in order to provide a vehicle for the patient's wisdom to inform clinical decision making.

Articulated in the specific language of the therapy, a basic pharmacoethological assessment follows this sequence of questions:

1. From what repertoire of social behavior will a solution need to come if a distressing symptom is to be alleviated? Steven was a pleasant 8-year-old boy who took apart my office in 10 minutes, shredding my fig tree of its leaves. Uncertain whether his drivenness and distractability were context dependent, I also observed him at school, where he had to sit next to the teacher's desk, because he could neither sit still nor finish tasks. His parents, his teacher, and I could agree, with no need for more technical language, that he needed to be able to focus his attention if he were to be able to pass his schoolwork and to have enjoyable relationships with parents and friends.

2. Which emotional postures provide the patient with access to this repertoire of social behavior? Can the patient easily access these emotional postures? Is the problem a general lack of access to emotional postures of tranquility? Is the problem one of dominance by a particular emotional posture

that excludes alternatives? Like many children diagnosed with attention deficit disorder, Steven was literally unable to ignore sights and sounds around him; he could not habituate to irrelevant events in his life-world. In terms of emotional posture, he could not leave an exploratory posture, in which his attention was maximally attuned to notice any novel event in the environment. In order to function, he needed emotional postures of tranquility in which he could reflect quietly or could hold selective attention for his task at hand.

3. If these emotional postures can be accessed only with difficulty, or not at all, can this access be enhanced by reattuning brain systems for regulating emotional postures? Neurophysiologically, focused attention is enabled by circuits that integrate the reticular formation (a core meshwork of brain systems that we share with amphibians, reptiles, and birds) and the prefrontal cortex (an outermost brain structure that is elaborated extensively only in humans). Although animals with well-developed systems within the reticular formation possess excellent attention for stalking, such as cats that watch birds or frogs that watch flies, only the integration of reticular formation systems with prefrontal cortex systems permits the adjustment and shifting of attention with language, as when we are instructed by others or by our own self-talk to pay careful attention to completing a task. Although a person can fail to learn to use the available attentional capacity of the brain, a child with severe, pervasive attentional problems, such as Steven, more often seems to have structural problems somewhere in the reticular formation-prefrontal cortex circuitry (Zametkin et al., 1990).

4. If brain systems can be reattuned, which brain systems are they, and what are the processes of reattunement? The efficiency of the reticular formation-prefrontal cortex circuits is in turn regulated by the dopamine system, a cousin to the norepinephrine system that is also located at the base of the brain and also regulates behavioral states, albeit toward different ends. The dopamine system helps the nervous system keep matters of priority on front stage. It is somewhat analogous to the channel selector on a home-entertainment center that permits one to listen to the CD player, to watch television, or to listen to FM radio, depending on which switch is turned on. It facilitates shifts among multiple brain systems that are processing different kinds of information concurrently, enabling information of greatest priority to dominate attention.

The easiest method for tuning attention is by adjusting the dopamine system activation with medications. Stimulant drugs prime the dopamine system, enhancing focused attention. This is an effect of the amphetamine family of drugs upon normal individuals, not just those with attention problems, as college students learn each spring when taking Dexedrine to study for exams. In addition to the amphetamines, such as Dexedrine, there are some other stimulants that also have an acceptable degree of dopamine-stimulating efficacy in boosting focused attention (Committee on Children with Disabilities, 1987; Zametkin et al., 1990).

In some clinical situations, such as Steven's, the problem and the medications are each well-enough understood that their interfacing can be made logically and coherently. Steven's behavior and performance at school improved remarkably after taking a stimulant medication, and I no longer feared his visits to the office, no doubt a therapeutic effect on our relationship, too.

Unfortunately, there are other clinical situations in which we are limited in how far we can go in a similar sociophysiological analysis of a patient's problem. Our understanding of how neurophysiology and social behavior are related is still primitive. In recent years psychopharmacologists, in a zeal for research grant support, and pharmaceutical companies, in a zeal for profits, each have tended to overstate to the public the extent of our understanding, both for the brain mechanisms of the drugs clinicians use and for the meaning these mechanisms have in the natural world of a person's life. Often, as in a number of examples presented in this book, a clinician's use of medications is limited to attempting to facilitate a nonspecific shift from emotional postures of mobilization to those of tranquility. Yet, this is enough for many patients, for whom the careful use of medications can decide the difference between therapeutic success and therapeutic failure.

In years to come, the sophistication of this kind of pharmacoethological assessment will expand enormously, as we better understand mammalian social behavior among humans and as we ask pharmacological questions that center less on the psychological and neurochemical events within an isolated individual and more on what these events mean within the patient's social world.

Rendering Expert Knowledge Usable for Patients and Families Who Collaborate in Treatment

Medication treatment developed out of a hierarchical medical tradition, in which patients were expected to accept, passively and unquestioningly, their treatment as prescribed by a physician. With Steven, for example, some pediatric psychopharmacologists would have evaluated him, made a diagnosis of attention deficit disorder, and prescribed a stimulant to treat the disorder. Learning the family's language about the problem, helping the parents to understand how the medication seems to work within the nervous system, relating this understanding to new possibilities in Steven's social world, integrating social effects of the medication with therapeutic actions by the teacher and family members, constructing with the parents and teacher ways for assessing outcome—all would be seen as permissible actions for a clinician to take but not central to the treatment. Instead, the two primary goals of treatment would have been, first, a decrease in Steven's distractability and hyperactivity as judged by the clinician, and, second, "medication compliance," consisting of good documentation that Steven indeed was taking his medication.

The language of medicine, including that of medical psychiatry, is largely a language of patient compliance. With a minimal role for collaboration in the medical language tradition, a clinician must take active steps to convert the technical, expert knowledge about medication treatment into usable knowledge for patients and their families. This is less a requirement for patient education than it is a requirement for making transparent and understandable the technical processes that have evolved in formulating pharmacological treatments. Just as a reflecting team makes transparent the perceptual and cognitive processes of clinicians who work in therapy with language, a similar deconstruction of decision-making processes is needed for medication treatment, so that patients and family members understand how to participate in them (Griffith & Griffith, 1992a): The following are useful guidelines.

1. It is helpful to operationalize clinical decision making, because this renders public the private processes of judgment and reasoning employed by a clinician. For example, I (JLG) have spoken the following sentences many times when meeting with a patient to determine whether medication would be helpful for depression: "Psychiatrists who developed medication treatments for depression have used the term 'depression' somewhat differently from the manner in which it is used in everyday conversation. They use 'depression' to indicate not so much how someone feels inside but whether there is a particular pattern of bodily symptoms present on a daily basis. The questions I just asked you came from a Hamilton Depression Scale, which is considered to be the gold standard for predicting whether someone will benefit from antidepressants (Hamilton, 1960). Although only you can tell me whether or not you feel depressed, it turns out that the Hamilton Scale is a reliable indicator for whether your depression will respond to medications or not. Research has suggested that it is not so much the story of a person's life and how it led into depression that predicts whether medication will help as simply whether particular symptoms are present persistently in a particular pattern. The questions on the Hamilton Scale, such as those about sleep, appetite, energy, libido, are the questions that seem to be most important. That is, if 100 people who score 20 or more on the Hamilton Scale are given antidepressant medication, about 70 of them will score in the nondepressed range a month later."

Used in a collaborative, nonobjectifying manner, such standardized scales as the Hamilton Scale can be quite helpful in deconstructing clinical judgment, because they make visible a clinician's cognitive processes that otherwise would remain hidden.

2. It is also important to contextualize expert knowledge, rather than stating it as objective fact. Consider the difference between the following two statements: (1) "Drug Y is the drug-of-choice for treating depression"; and (2) "When a large group of patients who scored above 20 on a Hamilton Depression Scale—as you did—were given Drug Y, an average of 70% of them had their Hamilton Depression Scale scores drop by one-half. The others did not show much change. About 15% of the whole group found they could not take Drug Y because of unpleasant side effects."

When knowledge in placed in the historical context of its process of generation, persons of average intelligence can employ their wisdom from everyday experiences to use the knowledge effectively. When knowledge is pronounced ex cathedra, however, they cannot. Those who have played baseball, lived on a budget, sought advice from an accountant, or parented a child have the wisdom to judge whether and how to employ medication treatment if its language of description is in the everyday tongue.

3. It is helpful to collaborate with patients and family members in customtailoring outcome measures to determine whether treatment is accomplishing what was intended. "If we looked 2 months from now and this medication had helped in all the ways it could help, what would be different then? Who would notice? What would you see? What would be the smallest amount of change that would make a difference? How will we judge whether to continue the treatment?"

4. Patients and families find it difficult to participate effectively in a therapy in which the language used and the choices to be made are not congruent. Metaphors create stories about reality. Once a decision has been made about which therapies to pursue—pharmacological therapy, conversational therapy, or both—it is important that the language of the problem fit the therapies selected for its solution.

Coupling Language-Based and Physiology-Based Interventions through Metaphor

Every metaphor contains within it implicit, unstated assumptions about what is real and what is not. A metaphor selects a particular reality for those who employ it in their communications with others (Griffith, Griffith, Meydrech, Grantham, & Bearden, 1991).

Some metaphors that clinicians use create a reality in which a therapeutic conversation about a problem is the most sensible way to go about solving it. In such a reality, it might make no sense at all to try to change physiology with medications. Ellen Whitney, for example, was tormented by her guilt from an extramarital affair that had occurred 20 years earlier. It made no difference that her anxiety and depression scores on standardized rating scales were extraordinarily high. The root metaphor of her story was that of "penance"; her agitation was a just penance for her betrayal of her husband. Such a metaphor leaves no room to consider pharmacological treatment of her symptoms. Indeed, taking medications would be experienced by her as a sinful effort to escape life's moral order.

Other metaphors create a reality in which changing physiology with medications makes sense, but talking about the problem does not. Jack Henry, with a psychopharmacology text under his arm, came requesting medications for his "panic disorder." I (JLG) quickly learned that he, in fact, had been through prior courses of treatment with several other psychiatrists and that he already had taken all the commonly used regimens for panic anxiety in high doses for lengthy periods. A family meeting revealed that Jack was the son of a competitive, highly successful businessman. The father worked hard to avoid expressing the disgust he felt for Jack, who he saw as drifting through life, neither completing an education nor mastering a vocation. The family stories and communications validated Jack's picture of himself as living under high expectations, but with no competence for meeting those expections, an ideal psychological context for inviting panic. But Jack's core metaphor was that of "symptom capture," a term he learned from reading the psychiatric literature. He was on a never-ending search to find the drug that would "capture" his symptoms. The reality created by such a metaphor left no option for working with the relationship ecology of his symptoms.

A metaphor is an exclusionary metaphor if it brings into being a reality in which a domain of actions, whether conversational therapy or pharmacological therapy, has no logical place in the solution of the problem (Griffith et al., 1991). One of the widely used exclusionary metaphors that clinicians employ is a description of symptoms as a disease, or a "chemical imbalance." Jill Taylor, for example, was a 34-year-old woman who had completed three sessions of couples therapy with her husband, because their sexual relationship was unsatisfactory for each. Her therapist, thinking that depression might contribute to her low level of interest in sex, suggested that she obtain psychiatric consultation to determine the possible need for an antidepressant. The psychiatrist she saw agreed that she was depressed. Her lack of sexual desire, he told Jill, was part of a "chemical imbalance" in her brain that needed an antidepressant to be put right. Upon hearing this explanation, however, John, her husband, refused to attend further couples sessions, as "the problem was obviously in Jill's brain."

Other exclusionary metaphors that enjoy wide usage among clinicians are as follows.

1. Misbehavior metaphors. Some structural and strategic family therapists have sought behavioral change by reframing a psychiatric or medical symptom as a covert form of irresponsibility (Haley, 1980; Madanes, 1981). A clinician meeting with two parents about their depressed adolescent might say

to them, "I'm not sure what you mean when you say he is depressed, but I do see that he does not keep his room clean, is not studying enough to pass, and spends most of his day watching television." If accepted by the parents, this reframing of the problem can provide a fulcrum from which structural changes might be made in the habitual patterns of behavior in the family. But if this fails, it leaves no plausible role for antidepressant medications as an alternative.

2. Family game metaphors. Some systemic models for therapy have viewed the patient and family as a closed cybernetic system, within which each person's moves, like moves in a game, are consistent with the family rules (Fisch, Weakland, & Segal, 1983; Papp, 1983; Selvini, Palazzoli, Boscolo, Cecchin, & Prata, 1978). In such a rule-driven game, the symptom is simply another move in the game. A clinician, from this perspective, might say to a family whose teenage daughter has disabling headaches, "I am worried that your daughter's headaches may improve. If she were to feel well enough to become more interested in her high school friends and dating boys, less interested in the family relationships, and seldom at home, then the two of you might become more mindful of your unhappiness with each other, which could even threaten the marriage. For the sake of the family's stability, it is important—for the present—that your daughter continue to have headaches." In the recoiling from such a paradoxical intervention, the systemic therapist would hope that a social context contributing to the headaches would be disabled. However, it is difficult to incorporate pharmacological treatment coherently into such an intervention.

3. Addiction metaphors. The late 1980s were characterized by a resurgence of 12-step models of therapy based on AA's tradition for treatment of addiction. Clinicians began 12-step programs not only for persons addicted to alcohol and drugs but also for anorexia, bulimia, obesity, depression, gambling, and compulsive promiscuity. A clinician might approach a woman with bulimia with the message, implicitly or explicitly: "The fact that your binging and purging continue uncontrolled shows that you have not yet confessed your powerlessnes over your bulimia, nor have you really turned it over to your higher power." Although such an approach has been of enormous benefit to some patients, it has not been found useful by others. When it is less than fully successful, it is difficult to find a rational role for medications within the model, even though there are numerous studies showing the efficacy of pharmacological treatment of bulimia for selected patients.

For each of these exclusionary metaphors, implicit assumptions preclude either conversational or physiological solutions for the problem. There are, however, inclusionary metaphors, termed coupling metaphors, that create expansive realities within which physiological problem solving with drugs and conversational problem solving with language can easily coexist (Griffith et al., 1991). Coupling metaphors contain implicit assumptions that validate both conversational and physiological solutions for a problem. Examples of coupling metaphors include the following.

1. Stress-diathesis metaphors. It is assumed that there is an underlying physiological vulnerability for illness that becomes manifest only when the body is in an emotional posture of extreme mobilization. Such an assumption underlies the enormous quantity of research in the 1980s studying expressed emotion and its relationship to psychiatric symptoms (Goldman, 1988; Hogarty et al., 1986). From this perspective, a clinician might say to the parents of a patient who has recently been psychotic: "Nowadays, psychiatrists don't think of schizophrenia so much as a disease as a kind of learning disability for emotions. Your daughter may be able to do much of what she desires to do socially, but not with as much speed or intensity. If your daughter takes her time, can avoid high-performance pressures, and can learn to clear up conflict quickly in her personal relationships, then she is more likely to enjoy her life. But if she is pressed, or pressures herself, to perform above her capacity, or if she is deluged by uncertainty or frustration, her brain systems for processing information are likely to be overwhelmed, and she may begin hallucinating again. She can raise her threshold for tolerance of stress by taking Trilafon [an antipsychotic drug], but this may do little good unless we all work together in creating an optimal emotional environment."

2. Psychophysiological metaphors. Even the healthiest of bodies shows signs of illness if stressed too much for too long. The notion of a psychosomatic symptom, a legacy from psychoanalytic thought, is so much a part of our culture that no one is surprised if a headache, a duodenal ulcer, chest pains, or cramping muscles prove to have more to do with emotional events than with a primary disease state.

Recent research studies suggest an interpretation of severe depression as a state of chronically heightened vigilance and excessive emotional arousal. Such scientific interpretation, operationalized within the therapeutic dialogue, might lead a clinician to say to the depressed partner in a couple: "Perhaps you have been under so much emotional stress for so long that your brain systems for processing emotional stress are depleted. An antidepressant medication might be able to restore their chemical stores to a normal baseline. But you would need to work hard in therapy to create a life together in which the emotional demands on your body are in keeping with what your body was designed to meet when it was created." According to the metaphor, there would be a logical place, and perhaps necessity, for both conversational and pharmacological therapies.

3. Physiological adaptation metaphors. Ethologically minded clinicians have drawn convincing parallels between commonly occurring psychiatric symptoms among humans and comparable social behaviors among animals.

For example, depression can be likened to hibernation, in which the bodies of bears and alligators physiologically shut down in the face of a too harsh environment; a panic attack may be homologous to the drowning reflex; a conversion symptom may be homologous to the immobility reflex or "freeze reaction" that occurs when an animal is trapped; the rituals and compulsions of obsessive-compulsive disorder may be homologous to nesting behaviors. To the extent that such comparisons are valid, they point to a physiological adaptation of the body to a particular social context. It would make sense then to combine giving a pill to change the sensitivity of adaptation (e.g., by taking a pill, a bear might gain a few extra winter days before feeling it necessary to search for a hollow tree where he could retire) with using language to create a less harsh social world that would not trigger physiological withdrawal.

4. Domains-of-discourse metaphors. White and Epston (1990) employed the social analyses of such philosophers as Michel Foucault to identify domains of social discourse that wield power over the minds and bodies of persons who live within them. For White and Epston, such distinctions as "physiological" and "psychological" describe languages that organize social practices and self practices of those who accept and use the language. They are "language games," rather than representations of a reality beyond human experience (Hartnack, 1965). This distinction is significant, because it counters a commonly held assumption of our scientific culture that all psychological and social experiences ultimately are reducible to patterns of brain events within the involved persons.

Operationalized in a clinical setting, this perspective might lead a clinician to ask: "When the family is stressed, how much of it seems to come from the schizophrenia and how much from 'bad habits' that the schizophrenia may have initiated? Which parts do the medications help and which parts do they not? When schizophrenia dominates the life of your family, what positive aspects of you as a family does it hide? Can you tell me about your daughter as you know her as a person, in aspects that have nothing to do with schizophrenia? Are there some times when she controls the influence of the schizophrenia? How does she do this?"

These questions contain an implicit, unstated assumption that schizophrenia is a problem brought into being by a scientific language of psychiatry along with prescribed social practices for its remediation, such as the taking of antipsychotic medications. Although such questions do not undermine the usefulness of the scientific story, they implicitly point out that the scientific story cannot fully account for the patient's and family's experience of distress and that it is not fully sufficient for a solution.

White and Epston (1990) use discourse-dividing language to demarcate a circumscribed problem domain for schizophrenia, set apart from other domains of life that it can intrude on but can never fully incorporate. By

implication, medications have their place within the schizophrenia discourse, but other healing practices would fit best other domains of discourse.

The Difficulty of Coordinating Pharmacological and Conversational Therapies

The integration of conversational therapy with pharmacological therapy can
be difficult at times. A primary difficulty arises from the fact that conversational (narrative) and physiological descriptions of problems are alternative
descriptions that cannot be reduced or translated one into the another. One
man, relating a life story of failure, loss, and incompetence, becomes listless
and depressed, with fitful sleep, no appetite, and no interest in sex. Another
man, taking a blood-pressure medication that alters his brain chemistry,
shows an identical set of depression symptoms, even though the circumstances of his life are pleasurable and rewarding. One man's depression is
described in terms of dreams, choices, and disappointments; the other in
terms of brain depletion of its catecholamine neurotransmitters. Neither
man's problem would be understandable in the other man's language; yet, a
clinician is presented only with depression symptoms and a request to
relieve the suffering. Which kind of treatment should be used, or should it
be both? If treatments of unlike kind are randomly combined, like a potluck
supper where no one is told what to bring, the combined efficacy of multiple
treatments can be less than that of either used alone.

The key to escaping this dilemma is found in the dual definition ascribed
to an emotional posture: An emotional posture is both an embodied self-narrative and a physiological state of the body. This dual description provides a
juncture between language and physiology that enables us to understand
conversational and pharmacological change as related through structural
selection (Chiari & Nuzzo, 1988).

Structural selection describes a kind of relationship through which events
in phenomenal domains that do not intersect can nevertheless influence one
another. Events occurring in the linguistic domains of a person's life, conversations, self-talk, arguments, admonitions, do not dictate specific physiological states, but they do limit or expand possiblities that certain physiological states will occur. Likewise, physiological events, the body states
belonging to hunger, sexual arousal, sleepiness, rage, do not dictate specific
conversations or relationships, but they do limit or expand possibilities that
particular conversations and relationships will occur. We can thus discuss
how critical self-narratives select for the body a repertoire of physiological
states that are permitted to occur, and how physiological changes in brain
information-processing systems select a repertoire of self-narratives through
which one's life-world can be experienced. An emotional posture is the

expression of this mutual specification of the body by story and by brain.

Structural selection offers a way of understanding mind-body relationships that avoids the traps of traditional philosophical positions, such as idealism, materialism, dualism, or interactionism. From this perspective, the questions in a conversational therapy and the medications in a pharmacological therapy each bias the frequency of occurrence of therapeutically desirable emotional postures.

The Limits of Pharmacological Treatment

Pharmacological treatment, like every other therapy, presents certain problems that arise with regularity because of the structure of the therapy. As such, they can be minimized but not always avoided. Two such problems for pharmacological therapy are the loss of a sense of personal agency that can occur in some treatment contexts, and the risk of self-objectification when pharmacological treatment becomes an effort to gain instrumental control over one's body.

Medications and Personal Agency

For many, taking a medication evokes images of weakness, loss of responsibility, and submission to medical authorities. Historically, these are attributions that have closely accompanied the sick role in Western culture. These associations can invite an emotional posture of submission that obscures a patient's awareness of life choices, to the patient's detriment.

Sarah came to see me (MEG) to prepare herself to attend a business meeting that was required by her company. She read to me from her journal to let me know how bad it was. "I am terrified when I think about having to go to that meeting with 20 people in a room with a door closed. I would rather face someone with a loaded gun in a deserted parking lot late at night with nobody else around. I have racked my brains, but I can't think of a way out of it. There are no words to express how scared I feel."

Because she seemed to talk with me with such ease, I inquired about the source of her dread. "It's the men—I can't stand to be with men in a closed room. I get hot, I break out in a cold sweat, my heart starts pounding, I feel like I'm going to faint. The only way I can survive is to keep my head down and never to look up at them." As she told the stories of her relationships with an abusive father and abusive partners earlier in her life, her dread began to make sense. I wondered how she had managed to leave these men.

She told the story of fleeing from Tom, the abusive partner, in the middle of the night and establishing an independent life for herself. She wanted never to have to rely on a man again. In fact, she had not even had an extended conversation with a man for several years. But now her distancing from men was hindering her advancement at work. Still, when she thought of the interactions she would have to have with men, she felt frightened and embarrassed, and the panic symptoms would start again. We worked in therapy on the voices she heard of men from the past—her father and Tom shaming and threatening her if she stood up for herself—and of her hearing her own strong, clear voice.

After a few sessions I suggested a medication consultation. I told her there might be a medication that could quiet her body's noisy alarm system, so that she could hear her own voice and could act on its wisdom. With an antianxiety medication, Xanax, she was able to go to the business meeting. Not only did she sit through it, she sat next to some men and conversed.

SARAH: Xanax took me to the meeting, and now it's going to get me a promotion! Now I can advance in my job and do the work I am capable of doing. I've been sitting so long in that position just because I couldn't talk to men. It is amazing what that Xanax is doing for me! I hope I never lose it.

MEG: Wait! I know the Xanax helps, but what did it do, and what did you do?

SARAH: Xanax did all of it! I'd have been under the table . . . fainted . . . on the floor.

MEG: Okay, so, it kept you from fainting. As you were then able to sit at the table, what did you do?

SARAH: Well, I talked to the man beside me. I did that. In fact, it was when I talked to him that I decided I could go talk to my boss.

MEG: Wow! What was it you noticed about yourself while you were talking to that man that told you that you could talk to your boss?'

SARAH: That I made good sense. . . . He noticed it, then I noticed it. He was really interested in my ideas. See, I have good ideas about what the company can do. In fact, I have more ideas than most people, because I have collected them in storage for so long. [We laughed.]

MEG: So you had them in storage, and you just had to open the door?

SARAH: Well, the Xanax opened the door.

MEG: Okay. Then, when the door was opened, did the Xanax bring out the ideas, or did you?

We bantered on playfully for a while. Then we talked seriously about how she had suffered from panic attacks all these years. She told about the decision points of her life: the decision to go to vocational training to become financially independent, rather than to stay at home; the decision to take the risk of leaving Tom, instead of to cower; the decision to move to a larger office despite her dread, rather than to stay in a smaller office with lower pay. There were many stories of her taking charge of her life, facing danger and dread, and facing them down—all before Xanax. Now the Xanax could be a welcome addition to her actions, but not the actor.

Self-Objectification by Seeking Instrumental Control over One's Body through Medications

Martin Heidegger many decades ago warned about the destructiveness of a scientific hubris that only seeks prediction and control over the natural world, at the expense of understanding relationships within the natural world. Heidegger warned that a radical objectification of the life-world by science would give rise to a radical "subjectivism" in how the fruits of science would be put to use (Palmer, 1969, pp. 144–145).

One trouble that can be visited on patients represents the fruition of Heidegger's warning. The elegance and sophistication of pharmaceutical research has been extraordinary during this century. It has promised to free patients from symptoms, such as pain, depression, and anxiety, that have oppressed humans since the dawn of our history. But the conduct of this research has been to focus narrowly on isolating chemicals that can manipulate in powerful ways isolated physiological and psychological variables, such as mood, sleep, or arousal, with little effort to understand the implications for the whole of a person's life and relationships if one such variable is so tightly controlled.

For many patients, there is no overarching wisdom to guide how such medications fit within the whole of one's life. Consequently, medications for some have come to mean trading a new, and sometimes worse, oppressor for the old. The worst scenario is one of addiction, in which a patient, trying to escape pain and suffering, as with narcotics, or trying to find pleasure and ecstasy, as with cocaine, becomes caught in an out-of-control cycle of escalating drug use for diminishing drug effects, until his or her whole life is organized around seeking the drug.

Most medications used in psychiatry have little or no risk for physiological addiction, compared to narcotics or crack cocaine. Few could be sold profitably on street corners by drug dealers. Nevertheless, patients can become bound by the same ideas as those that entrap persons in bona fide addictions. Chief among these is a failure to heed one of the most valuable lessons in cybernetics that was taught by Gregory Bateson (1972): In living systems, any effort to control rigidly one isolated part of a whole system inevitably destabilizes other regions of the system. Put in our context, one who seeks to control the body instrumentally with medications in order to avoid at all costs a specific type of distress is at risk for finding chaos and suffering in life as a whole.

This is perhaps the best way to understand the suffering of Jack Henry, who felt that he could not bear a particular kind of pain that arose especially in relationship to his father and his father's expectations. Medications from psychiatrists he consulted—imipramine, phenylzine, fluoxetine, alprazo-lam—each brought some relief, but none could banish the panic entirely. The harder Jack pressed his medications to guarantee him an anxiety-free life, the more impoverished and disorganized his life became. As his father's frustration over his increasing nonproductivity grew, it became a source of anxiety that could override any stabilization his medications had provided.

How does a clinician help patients to stay free of this trap? Several guide-lines have been helpful for us:

1.) A clinician can avoid promising too much. It is reliably more productive if a medication is presented as able, optimistically, to reduce suffering by one-third to one-half. Other nonmedical healing practices, whether a relationship-focused therapy, change in life-style, or aerobic exercise, may further reduce the rest of it. The goal then is to render life liveable, not ideal.

2.) A clinician can avoid reductionistic explanations for problems. When a problem is defined solely as a physiological disorder, it is too hard not to engage in fantasies about drug miracles. In our culture, who could not marvel at the story of Fleming's serendipitous discovery of penicillin or Banting's against-the-odds discovery of insulin?

3.) A patient can work to develop an ongoing dialogue with his or her body that embodies acceptance and respect. Most often, wildly out-of-control problems such as that presented by Jack Henry are characterized by a monological, controlling, demanding inner conversation between the patient and his or her body. For example, "Stop it! Stop it! You're lazy! You disgust me!" had become a personal mantra for one bulimic teenager. Much of her therapy consisted of learning to accept and to feel compassion for her body, eventually learning to hear its words rather than a driven urge to binge food. Wise pharmacological practices can also appear when a patient, instead of debating it, learns how to listen, to reflect on, and to harken to the voice of his or her body.

The Training of Clinicians

Training clinicians to conduct pharmacoethological therapies as outlined here will require that significant revisions be made in professional training pro-grams in this nation. The most radical changes required would be those in the professional education for psychiatrists. Over the past 20 years, many psychia-trists have felt most proud of their profession as they have witnessed its "remedicalization," which is widely held as synonymous with the institution of the DSM-III (now DSM-IV) nosology and drug treatments for the syndromes DSM-III created. In like mind we also call for greater medical competence, a better understanding of basic pharmacological mechanisms of psychiatric drugs, and, specifically, a deeper understanding of neuroanatomy, neurophysiology, and ethology than psychiatrists of past generations gained in their educations. Yet, we also see the DSM-III and IV and the pervasive neurobiological reductionism in psychiatric education as serious obstacles to training clinicians who are competent. Only when competence in using language to create therapeutic conversations and therapeutic relationships becomes the centerpiece of psychiatric education will psychiatrists become clinicians able to use effectively the fruits of the pharmaceutical industry.

Professional training for clinicians who are neither nurses nor physicians has for too long avoided the physiology within which all human behavior is embodied. It is noteworthy that as 1992 ended, there were only half a dozen published articles in the major family therapy journals that focused on the joint use of pharmacological therapy and family therapy. This avoidance has too often left the door open for psychological and social reductionisms, in which a patient's or a family's problem is assumed to be fully explained and understood in terms of operant conditioning, the function of the symptom in the family, intergenerational loyalties, or preservation of organizational hierarchy. Such reductionisms are as impoverishing as neurobiological reductionism by psychiatrists. At their worst, they have led to destructive pathologizing of parents and families who have simply been doing the best they could do in hard and complicated situations.

If nonmedical training programs take seriously a physiological perspective of clinical symptoms, then clinical theories that exclude such a perspective will need to be omitted and other theories revised. Training program faculties will need to come to grips with how to enable graduate students who do not have nursing or medical training backgrounds to learn about aspects of neuroanatomy, neurophysiology, and pharmacology that provide an understanding of physiological explanations for human behavior.

In order to conduct the therapy presented here, both medical and nonmedical trainees will need to learn more about how to create consultative relationships with patients and families, rather than relying on the power of a hierarchical relationship to specify to patients and families how they should conduct their lives. Above all, learning how to use language to weave the knowledges and skills from multiple perspectives into a seamless therapy will need to be placed at the forefront of professional education.

CHAPTER 11

Using Language in the Treatment of Medical Illness

O VER LUNCH, a retired chairman from our Department of Medicine reminisced over the transformations that had taken place in medical treatment since he had been in residency training 40 years earlier. "Thyroid disease . . . when I was in medical school, somebody would come to the emergency room in a "thyroid storm," and we would know what had happened—there had been a fight at home." In the old days of medicine, physicians and nurses feared the sudden appearance of a patient in a thyroid storm, the often-lethal surge of hypermetabolism, with racing heart and rising temperature, that happened when an overactive thyroid gland suddenly dumped far too much hormone into the bloodstream. Little could be offered, except to try keep the body chilled and the patient alive, while drops of thiopropouracil and iodide—the inadequate but sole available treatment—took days to slow down the activity of the gland. Physicians were limited in the extent to which they could manipulate body physiology. But they had more of a sense that the sudden appearance of a disease, such as hyperthyroidism, did not happen out of the blue, but as part of the fabric of a patient's lived experience.

Today, no endocrinologist, if asked, would be perplexed that a marital fight, its aggression flooding the body with catecholamines, might trigger an unstable thyroid gland to overstep its regulation of body metabolism. But who would ever wonder about such a thing? Today, few doctors or nurses in the United States ever witness a thyroid storm. Patients with hyperthyroidism are identified quickly in an early stage of their disease by laboratory tests. The biomedical treatment of the disease, by medications and by surgery, is so effective that no one would ever imagine a need to explore how the pathophysiology of the disease interacts with the life events and experiences in a patient's life. Only the older clinicians remember the evidence that there is a connection.

The shift to a biomedical understanding of illness in medicine has been nearly completed in the late twentieth century, because so much knowledge and skill have accrued for manipulating the anatomy and physiology of the human body to stop disease. Most medical students do not even realize that there is a distinction between *illness*, what a patient experiences, and *disease*, what a diagnostician sees when viewing a patient through the lens of physical examinations and laboratory tests (Kleinman, 1988). Yet, strong evidence is available that few medical illnesses occur isolated from the life experience of the patient. Aside from widespread recognition that chronic medical diseases, such as Alzheimer's disease, fare best when the whole family is involved in treatment, the lay public and most clinicians agree that major medical illnesses, such as cancer, heart disease, and hypertension, are influenced by beliefs, attitudes, and emotions. Even appendicitis, an illness seldom regarded as anything other than an infectious and surgical disease, has an occurrence highly related to recent stressful life events (Creed, 1989).

Although the benefits of biomedical treatments are undeniable, the cultural practices their success has instilled both in the medical professions and among the lay public have had negative consequences. No one would recommend psychotherapy as preventive treatment for appendicitis, because antibiotics and surgery are so effective, but the same mind-set applied to heart disease, lung cancer, and AIDS have led us too long down the path of seeking answers from new drugs and surgeries, rather than the aggressive promotion of healthier styles of living.

The ideological conflict between biomedical and social views of illness today is played out in the treatment of chronic medical illnesses, such as AIDS, chronic obstructive pulmonary disease, cancer, end-stage renal disease, or cystic fibrosis. Because there is a well-defined disease and available pharmacological or surgical treatments, biomedical clinicians tend to overlook the influence of communication and personal relationships on the course of the illness. Recently, however, there has been a growing appreciation of these language-mediated influences on the course of medical illnesses, particularly when biomedical treatments can treat but cannot cure, as is usually the case with chronic medical illness.

Behavioral Scientists in Medicine

As the limitations of biomedical science became increasingly evident, there arose during the 1970s and 1980s a burgeoning interest among mental health professionals for showing that they can offer corrective changes that bio-medicine cannot, by redirecting attention toward personal health habits and social influences on illness. The field of behavioral medicine, occupied mostly by behavioral psychologists, concentrated on researching the influ-ence of life-style on health. They began by designing behavioral programs to stop smoking, to lose weight, to follow healthy diets, to reduce stress responses, to develop a routine of aerobic exercise. Specific diseases, such as hypertension, were targeted for research that would lead to behavioral methods for treating the medical illness.

At the same time, systemic family therapists were organizing a new disci-pline, family systems medicine, to study how health and family life were related and how medical treatment could be delivered in a family context. Family researchers studied a wide range of illnesses to determine relation-ships between health and such family variables as structure, problem solv-ing, worldview, and management of emotions (Campbell, 1986; Fisher, Ran-som, Terry, & Burge, 1992; Minuchin, Rosman, & Baker, 1978; Ransom, Locke, Terry, & Fisher, 1992; Wood et al., 1989). By the 1990s, increasing numbers of family therapists were practicing medical family therapy, in which a family therapist would collaborate with a primary care physician in the treatment of medical illnesses (McDaniel, Hepworth, & Doherty, 1992).

Language-Based Therapy and Medical Illness

The clinical approach presented here diverges from the dominant traditions of both medical family therapy and behavioral medicine in its reliance on the specific language and personal experience of patients and families. Some family therapists have incorporated an assessment of family beliefs into comprehensive therapies with the medically ill (Rolland, 1990), and nurse-family therapists have specifically focused on changing family beliefs that impair health and hinder healing from illnesses (Wright & Leahy, 1987). But most family therapists and family researchers have focused on variables other than personal interpretations by patients and family members of their life experience.

These approaches can be described as etic in their epistemology, in that they study patient and family behavior in order to describe its patterns according to observer-defined criteria. By contrast, emic approaches are based on descriptions drawn from categories of meaning belonging to the people under study, the "folk perspective." (Pelto & Pelto, 1978; Taylor & Bogdan, 1984). The terms etic and emic, as used by anthropologists, describe whether the external, scientific-observer perspective (etic) or the internal, "native" perspective (emic) is given greater privilege in defining a culture. From an etic perspective, an anthropologist observes the behaviors of members of a culture, describing them according to concepts that can be employed across cultures, preferably in quantitative, statistically analyzable terms. From an emic perspective, members of a culture are interviewed in their native language in order to discover the natives' original categories of meaning, with systems and cultural patterns identified by logical and linguistic analysis (Pelto & Pelto, 1978). With a few notable exceptions (Andersen, 1987; Anderson & Naess, 1986; Barlow et al., 1987; Epston, 1986), neither medical family therapy nor behavioral medicine has employed emic approaches that organize therapy primarily around patients' and family members' personal, historical narratives of their illness.

Without questioning the usefulness of contributions that etic approaches have made for the care of the medically ill, there are clinicial situations where the limitations of these approaches stand out. A majority of our requests for consultation by a physician are prompted by nonproductive dialogue between the physician and a patient or family. Sometimes, dialogue has broken down because of a dispute as to whether symptoms are arising from the disease or whether psychological and social factors are their main determinants. More often, the physician believes that the progress of treatment is hindered because the patient or the family are "noncompliant." Here an emic therapy fits well when etic therapies do not.

A Noncompliant Mother

Jawana, a 10-year-old girl, was lying comatose in the Pediatrics Intensive Care Unit (PICU). The PICU charge nurse had called me (MEG). "We are having a serious problem, and it seems to be getting worse instead of better as time goes on. There is a little girl who was brought to us—postencephalitic, comatose, severely brain-damaged [from a viral infection of the brain]. Her mother has been here, almost without breaks, for a month now. The nurses and doctors have been totally honest with her, but she still believes her child will recover. Aside from our own strain, we are afraid that the mother will collapse. Also, we will need the bed for other children. We have committed not to press this mother to take her to a nursing home before she is ready, but there is pressure to have the acute bed available. We see her suffering, but we just can't seem to communicate with her, and we thought maybe you could talk with her."

I went to the PICU that day and found Susan, a tall, strong, African-American woman, performing a passive range of motion exercises on her daughter. I started to introduce myself, to explain my presence, and to ask Susan to join me in the conference room. Earlier in my family therapy career, I might have pressed to talk with everyone at once—staff and family members. But the nurses said they wanted me to talk with the mother, then with them to help them to understand the mother. I accepted this role, since, as consultant, I believe it to be most respectful to enter the system by the door that is opened, if that does not so hinder the consultation that it is crippled. The stories can begin to be heard among a few people, then, often, that group can grow, and more stories will be told and heard. It is this focus on the value of the simple telling and hearing of personal stories that has freed me to greater flexibility in these situations.

I sensed a disinterest from Susan in having any conversation with me. Her eyes were on Jawana, which told me that I should first let Jawana be introduced to me. As I took her limp hand and spoke to her, I noticed that behind the oxygen mask her hair had been carefully braided and ribboned. I began to help Susan with the range of motion exercises.

"I am a nurse, also," I mentioned, offering my passport to what seemed to be sacred space.

"Oh?" she said, unimpressed and silent as we continued to exercise Jawana. Then she spoke, "But . . . are you a mother?" She looked up and met my eyes for the first time. Her direct gaze told me she knew the answer to this question.

"Yes," I answered. I silently wondered if she had known that when I had touched her daughter, imagining her more alive and playing, that my thoughts had wandered to my own child playing and suddenly being struck down. Could she have known?

"Yes, and I also have a 10-year-old. I can't imagine what this is like for you. You must be very tired."

Susan then carefully tucked Jawana in and invited me into the conference room. I knew that I was invited on the terms of my being a mother, not primarily as a nurse or family therapist.

"I am tired, but I'm not sad, not today anyway. And they can't understand that. I guess if they called you, they think I'm crazy."

"No," I explained, "They are worried about you, that you work with Jawana so hard and so long that you will become exhausted. They are worried that they can't communicate with you."

Susan did not believe that any of the nurses or doctors understood her. She wondered, in fact, if they were capable of understanding, because her knowledge was from the Lord and theirs was just from science. I asked if there were any nurses who understood at all.

"Betty Ann. I believe Betty Ann understands," pointing to an African-American nurse who was caring now for Jawana. "She is the one who fixed up Jawana's hair in that pretty way."

I was relieved that there appeared to be multiple, more complex, descriptions of the system organized around Jawana than that which I had first been told in the initial consultation.

"Could I understand better if Betty Ann would join us?" I asked. Susan expressed pleasure at the suggestion. Betty Ann was an LPN—a licensed practical nurse—hierarchically at a lower level among the caregivers.

Joining us, Betty Ann smiled, "Jawana and I are big buddies . . . and Susan, too." They both laughed comfortably together and talked as friends. Betty Ann recalled when she had been in a family caregiver role when her own mother had been critically ill.

This open disclosure of Betty Ann's personal life and the comradery she had with Susan would have been disapproved according to many definitions of nursing professionalism, just as my disclosure about being a mother would have been disapproved by my psychotherapy supervisors during training. But Susan, surrounded by professionals, with her child's life in the balance, obviously wanted to entrust herself only to those who could show themselves to be ordinary people.

I asked Betty Ann to describe her understanding of the PICU staff's concerns. "It is true," she said, "They don't understand Susan's faith. But all of us are worried about her fatigue. We know she loves Jawana and wants her to know her mama is near. But we wish she would let us help her out a little more."

My role was that of a facilitator in this conversation, asking these women about their thoughts about the problem, then what experiences in their lives had led them to these thoughts. I asked each woman about her imaginings about Jawana's future.

Susan said she believed God was going to heal her. God had given her this hope through a dream. When I asked whether she ever entertained doubts, she said that she had doubts, but then God gave her the dream a second time, this time even more clearly. Also, she listed many subtle signs of improvement in Jawana that she had seen but that the nurses and doctors either could not see or would not admit to seeing "because they don't want to raise my hopes."

Betty Ann said, "To us, it doesn't look good or hopeful for Jawana, but you never know what God will do." She agreed she had seen some of the signs Susan had witnessed and not others. "But," she told Susan, "Sometimes you can see things we can't see, physically and spiritually." Susan looked relaxed. This seemed to be a good ending place, so we parted.

Susan left the hospital later that day for a rest. The nurses were pleased that she had relaxed enough to leave and asked me to return. I kept in touch with Susan over the ensuing days. She was visiting home more often to attend to her other daughter. But on the 10th day she told me, "I'm outnumbered. The PICU people are working toward Jawana's staying just like she is or even trying to get me ready to lose her. I'm getting her ready for when she will walk again."

Susan didn't want to meet with the staff but wanted me to talk with them. "She's right," her pediatrician said. "While we don't want to be brutal, we can't be dishonest or encourage her denial. And we have questions that must be answered about her life-support systems and her long-term care. If she stays alive, she belongs in a long-term care facility, not an intensive care unit. ... I have learned to always say, 'never say never,' but we know this child will not improve. We have to deal with the questions we have with the mother. We need to meet together. Do you think she would meet us with you?" If Betty Ann were present, I answered, it might be possible.

Mindful of the constraints, I had two thoughts about how to create a conversational domain adequate for this meeting. First, if the conversation were to feel unsafe to Susan, it would feel unsafe because she would feel it to be unbalanced. Second, I felt that the disparate views on Jawana's future and its pressing questions had compelled us to look only in the present and the future. I hoped that stories from the past could provide us with a better meeting place where we could talk.

Remembering Susan's words, "I'm outnumbered here," I asked her which persons might best understand and support her. Who would she most want to have by her side? In addition to Betty Ann, she wanted to invite Jawana's grandmother—Susan's ex-mother-in-law—and Susan's ex-husband, who had shown little involvement until then. As a former intensive care unit nurse and now a preacher in her church, the grandmother could speak clearly and with authority.

We gathered, and before I could even "start the session," the air filled with stories of which I had been unaware. "Oh yes, I remember this hospital," said Jawana's grandmother. "This is where Susan's cousin, Minnie, had her baby. Minnie was bleeding, and was so ill. It wasn't time for the baby, and they thought she'd lose it. They called all the family to come and to pray. They especially called me, knowing I'd lost children of my own and could comfort her the way only an older woman can. So she delivered the baby—such a small thing. The doctors knew right away that it wouldn't live, and it did stop breathing. They put the baby up on the cold counter and brought us the death certificate. But before I went to comfort Minnie, God told me to look at the baby. "This baby's alive!" I hollered. It was breathing and squirming! I picked her up off that cold counter and warmed her in my arms."

At this moment, the faculty pediatrician paled. "Yes, I was there! I was an intern. The baby was dead, or so we thought. It's true—we had started a death certificate. I've never been so surprised in my life. In fact, *that* baby is why I always say 'never say never.' So that's *your* granddaughter? How is she?"

"Oh, she's fine." the grandmother said. "She's a tiny girl, but she's smart and likes to read and to sing and to play with Jawana. In our family we know about miracles."

"Wow! Do you mean there are other miracle stories?" I asked.

The grandmother then told about a time she thought her son was dead but he was alive. He had been in a terrible wreck and should have died but turned out to have been thrown safely into tall grass off the side of the road.

"Are there ever times when God has told you to let go of someone?" I asked.

"Yes," the grandmother replied, "When I was nursing my husband, God finally gave me a confirmation and let him go home. People didn't understand it then either, but I had absolute peace."

"The peace that passeth understanding," Susan spoke softly.

The pediatrician asked the questions that were facing them about Jawana's long-term care and her needed life-support systems. She added that the questions did not have to be answered now and assured Susan that her wishes would be respected. No plans would be implemented without her approval.

Both Susan and Jawana's grandmother indicated that if God were to give them confirmation that "she was not to be raised up," then they would want to discontinue her life support.

Jawana's father was less certain. "This is my only daughter," he said. "I just don't know if I can say that yet."

The conversation had shifted again. It appeared that the people who needed to talk together could talk, and now they talked more in terms of "yet" and "not yet," rather than "yes" or "no." The talk included stories of miracles told by all participants, of life being given back and of life being taken away. Different ways of knowing were acknowledged, from nursing, medical, spiritual, and cultural traditions, as well as the special knowledge only a mother can possess about her child.

My presence was no longer needed. I dropped by the PICU to visit Susan occasionally, but no formal consultations were requested thereafter, because there was effective communication between Susan and the staff. I later learned from Betty Ann that Susan had taken Jawana home and she had died there.

It is difficult to imagine how data from an empirical study about family structure and the chronically medically ill, or mothers with children in the ICU, or religious parents of comatose children, could have provided much guidance for either Susan, the ICU clinicians, or myself in resolving Susan's dilemma. Although a discussion among the clinicians that gave consideration to Susan's beliefs would, at the least, have enabled her interpreted experience to enter the planning of treatment, even that degree of objectification and exclusion from the discourse would likely have alienated her. The path to resolving Susan's impasse lay with building the kind of relationship and conversation in which each participant in the problem had a warrant to speak and would be heard in his or her own language. The unpredictable twists and turns through the conversation could never have been planned, but with care, skill, and respect, they could be followed.

An Intractable Case of Crohn's Disease

Biomedical clinicians often refer patients for psychiatric, psychological, or family consultations when it is evident that the outcome of medical treatment consistently falls short of expectations. Experienced physicians and nurses alert quickly to life stresses and to problems in relationships and communications, the so-called "psychosocial issues," when they account for a poor response to medical treatment.

When consulting to the treatment of a medical problem for which psychosocial issues are suspect, one asks: "What would constitute an optimal emotional environment for the healing of this patient's body?" Etic approaches have identified family structures, such as enmeshment; or problems in family development, such as an inability to make the transition from "family with small children" to "family with adolescent"; or specific behavioral sequences that prompt an exacerbation of the illness, such as an asthmatic child who starts wheezing when the parents argue. Once the type of family pathology has been identified, a clinician either educates the family about more adaptive styles of living that, according to research data, contribute to health, or introduces interventions directly to change dysfunctional behaviors or beliefs.

An emic approach also asks what the optimal healing environment would be, but from within the patient's experience using his or her narrative vocabulary, rather than the external observations of the scientific investigator. The clinician engages the patient and family members to inquire which emotions seem to precipitate or to intensify illness symptoms; what are the narratives from the patient's life story that are tightly connected to these emotional postures; which emotions seem to soothe the symptoms or hinder their occurrence; or what are the narratives from the patient's life story that are connected to these emotional postures. Techniques can then be employed that either reconstruct binding self-narratives or increase access to self-narratives that soothe the body or free its expression.

For example, a patient, Walter, was referred to me (JLG) for symptoms of Crohn's disease. His physician, when reaching the limits of what medications could offer for his bouts of pain, diarrhea, and constipation, asked that he seek psychiatric treatment in order to lessen the tenseness and anxiety that seemed to exacerbate his symptoms. In our meeting, we together identified a sense of "my guard is up" as a state of the body that was immediately associated with exacerbations of his symptoms. When "my guard is up" was dominant as his emotional posture, he was vigilant, body tensed, ready to run or fight. "My guard is up" seemed to stand for a bodily readiness to respond to an anticipated threat. Connected to it were "stories of failure"—being teased by larger boys while growing up, never feeling popular at school, confrontations with his parents whom he felt could never respect him.

When asked where in his life he found freedom from "my guard is up," he at first answered, "Only when I am 10 miles deep in the woods." He told how his body deeply relaxed only when he was so far away from any other human being that there was no possibility of any kind of human interaction. But when I persisted with close questioning, he did locate another place where this deep relaxation occurred in the presence of other people—when he attended his Alcoholics Anonymous (AA) group. When he was at AA he relaxed and felt "safe," a sensation he most experienced deep in his gut. "My whole gastrointestinal tract feels better." He described his AA meeting as the one place where he could speak openly with others about his most private fears, worries, and shame. Within the group there was an atmosphere of mutual acceptance without judgment. One could talk or remain silent; members spoke according to their own pace of comfort. Yet, there was a sense that value lay in sharing one's life story with the others, that pain involved in the telling would be redemptive and, with the other members' support, would be bearable. "In AA we have to be honest for ourselves and for others," he said.

In AA meetings and in his backpacking Walter could remove this camouflage, so that he and his compatriots could see what lay beneath. In time, he identified a few other occasions when, however briefly, he also felt this safety in his body. He connected these moments of safety—the forest, his AA meetings, the brief moments that had gone unnoticed—with parts of his life story he had not mentioned when we had first met: how he had held his job for 8 years despite his lack of education; how he earned his GED degree after dropping out of high school; how he had learned to hunt and fish and hike in the woods, even though no one had ever taught him how as a child. These were "stories of success." Together with life practices that he discovered were protective against his Crohn's disease symptoms, such as daily exercise, daily meditation, and avoidance of junk food and cigarettes, he also learned to access and to dwell within these stories of success in order to feel "safety" rather than "my guard is up."

The therapeutic work with Walter and similar patients lies mainly in techniques for freeing bodily expression. These methods include (1) identifying binding emotional postures; (2) identifying unspeakable dilemmas that bind bodily expression together with their associated self-narratives; and (3) learning how to escape these dilemmas, by disempowering the binding self-narratives and by accessing soothing self-narratives that free the body.

Embedding the Etic within the Emic

Etic and emic approaches have contrasting strengths and weaknesses in clinical situations. Etic approaches have proven most useful when patients and family members cannot distinguish usable patterns of illness and health in their experience of living. For example, there are family and social practices that adversely affect a person's health with a very long latency until illness, such as the production of lung cancer by smoking, or that is hidden from awareness during most of the course of the illness, such as the development of hypertension; or that follows very complex patterns of relationship, such as those proposed between "family enmeshment" and infant birth weight (Mengel, Davis, Abell, Baker, & Ramsey, 1991). When they are discerned, etic approaches can offer educational or training programs that facilitate health, much as an exercise physiologist can train an athlete in the most efficacious program for building muscle strength and endurance.

Emic approaches have been underused in the medicine of the late twentieth century. It has been slowly recognized that they offer their own strengths:

1.) Etic approaches rely on probabalistic reasoning from averaged measurements from large groups of patients. Therefore, it is never certain exactly how to apply them to the specific problem of a specific patient. Because emic approaches rely on the unique life story of the patient, they offer solutions that are clear and specific to a patient's problem.

2.) Etic approaches rely on education and instruction for their implementation. This immediately sets up a clinician-patient relationship based on compliance, in which the patient and family ought to defer to the expertise of the clinician. Because many requests for consultation arise in the first place because the patient or family is noncompliant with prescribed biomedical treatment, this is a serious problem for etic approaches. Emic approaches, on the other hand, rest on a collaborative relationship, in which treatment is cocreated by clinician and patient, thereby eliminating compliance as an issue.

3.) Families, not clinicians, are the primary caregivers for the chronically medically ill. Chronic medical illness therefore requires competent families. Reliance on the expert's special knowledge and skills in etic approaches secondarily devalues the competence of families. Emic approaches, however, take as a starting point the family's special knowledges and skills and build on them. Consequently, they enhance patients' and family members' sense of personal agency far more than do etic approaches.

4.) Etic approaches best describe in broad strokes the general patterns of symptoms in a particular illness. When a patient has a paroxysmal or rapidly fluctuating symptom or sudden exacerbation of a chronic symptom, such findings often are of little help in understanding the relationship between symptom occurrence and the idiosyncratic circumstances that triggered it. The explanations for symptom occurrences that an emic approach would gather from the patient and family members' observance of their daily life would be more likely to find specific and practical solutions.

Emic approaches, such as the language-based therapy we described, can contextualize and give new meaning to etic clinical approaches developed by family therapists, based on an understanding of family structure and family development. We each learned this lesson several years ago in a family therapy with the Henson family whose son, 15-year-old Billy, was critically ill with cystic fibrosis. Initially, Billy's pulmonologist sought a family consultation because of Billy's hypersensitivity to each new antibiotic that was tried for his lung infection. The pulmonologist felt satisfied that his reactions—rapid breathing, itching, breaking out in welts, fainting—had no physiological explanation, because they could be suppressed with injections of a placebo. However, they continued to be so severe that he could not tolerate the antibiotics. As his infection worsened, he was moved to the intensive care unit.

In a one-session consultation, I (MEG) met with Billy, his family members, and his pediatrician, attempting to understand the perspectives of each of these persons. The interview was transformative. Billy's reactions completely stopped, he received his antibiotics, and he was soon discharged from the hospital, again well. The outcome of the consultation was so dramatic that we published its description in a journal article (Griffith & Griffith, 1992b).

The story did not end there, however. Although Billy's hypersensitivity symptoms never returned, he and his family were still afflicted with all the distress that comes with severe, chronic medical illness. The family was financially overwhelmed by the costs of Billy's medical care and eventually exhausted the limits of their medical insurance. Billy's father had to work two jobs, and he became too absent from his home and marriage. Billy and his mother argued, and his sister received too little time and parental attention. When Billy became upset, it often triggered a crisis in his breathing.

At the time, the two of us often worked as cotherapists with difficult cases. Our clinical work was primarily developed out of structural and strategic systemic therapy. As a structural diagnosis, we assessed Billy's family as showing (1) mother-son enmeshment; (2) disengagement of the father; and (3) family conflict detoured through anxious attending to Billy's health needs. In addition, there were few signs that Billy's entry into adolescence had been accompanied by stage-appropriate developmental changes in family behavior that would encourage his autonomy, responsibility, and increased privacy within the family.

Based on this structural diagnosis and developmental assessment, we designed a myriad of interventions during three- to six-session therapies that occurred itermittently over the next few years. We gave the parents assignments to go on dates together, had the parents switch roles with father staying with Billy in the hospital, tried to provide respite for the parents by enlisting other persons in Billy's care, pressed for Billy to assume more responsibility and decision making in his medical treatment, encouraged more parental time with Billy's younger sister. The going was rough. Between-session assignments fizzled more often than not. The small changes achieved seldom persisted. Family members seemed to have barely enough will to go through the next day.

Despite what seemed to be minimal progress in achieving badly needed changes, the Hensons found our sessions useful enough to return. These meetings were infrequent, always occasioned by a family crisis around Billy's exacerbating symptoms. Every time, Mrs. Henson would say that she was ready again to "give him up" and encouraged Billy to let go, to let his suffering end, but Billy had no wish to let go. Billy's doctor felt that Billy was in charge of his own life and agreed to pursue the aggressive treatment Billy requested.

Mrs. Henson was aware that many staff and friends could not understand her attitude, and that some were even horrified. But she felt that her God had helped her to come to accept Billy's death, and that He wanted Billy whole and well, with Him in heaven.

We had known the Hensons for 5 years and had been meeting with them only on scattered occasions when we had our last visit. Billy was 20 years old. I heard that he was doing badly, near death, so I went by to see the family. Billy was comatose, and Mrs. Henson and I talked in the hallway outside his room. Very quickly she began to cry. "Twenty years. . . . It's just not fair! I was never prepared for this! If I had known he would see 20, maybe I could have handled the last 7 years better."

I was confused, but I listened on.

"The doctor told us when Billy was 5 years old, 'Love him now, you will never see his teenage years.' So then came Billy's 12th birthday, and I still believed the doctor. I didn't think that I could stand to give him up, so I prayed as hard as I could for him to get well. That wasn't going to be, though, so then I prayed to let go and, finally, God gave me peace. I could never forget them telling me that we would not see his teens, and when that peace came . . . I knew for certain that I was being prepared for his dying and that would be soon. But he fought it, and his 13th birthday came. We had to have it here in this hospital. We tried to anyway . . . this is no place for a birthday. I know I should have felt blessed to have him for some more time . . . and I tried! But then he would start suffering, hurting so bad, and it seemed we had only been given more time to suffer. He had good times in between, but I was struggling so much with this depression that I couldn't enjoy them. It was that way every year, every birthday, 14, 15, 16. . . . Why did they tell us that?"

I asked if she had ever brought it up with the doctors, or even with her husband or son. But she said that she had only talked about it with God, and found no lasting peace there, because she could not even trust God's peace when she felt it anymore.

Billy died 3 days after our conversation. Many questions have troubled me. Why had Mrs. Henson never told me this story? What liberating possibilities might it have opened up in Mrs. Henson's conversations with the doctors, her husband, her son, her God? How is it that it was spoken at the end of our relationship and not at the beginning?

One answer might be that it was only natural to listen to Mrs. Henson on that day. Any neighbor would know that this time, at the end of a life, is a time for listening, not for suggesting. As any good neighbor, I wanted to create an environment for listening to her story. However, it is also true that I was working differently by then in my clinical work. I had come to value the speaking and hearing of stories in a different way, to see them as foreground instead of background to a therapy, as in motion even as they are spoken.

The emic does not displace the etic, but it does transform it. The structural changes we sought for the family had value, as evidenced by experiences of other clinicians with families with chronic illnesses and by the Henson family choosing to return periodically to see us. But the language I had spoken was alien to their experience. I failed to learn their vocabulary of stories. How might therapy have gone differently if Mrs. Henson's story could have been spoken and understood years earlier?

References

AMERICAN PSYCHIATRIC ASSOCIATION. (1987). *Diagnostic and statistical manual of mental disorders* (3rd ed., rev.). Washington, DC: Author.

ANDERSEN, T. (1987a). The general practitioner and consulting psychiatrist as a team with "stuck" families. *Family Systems Medicine, 5,* 468–481.

ANDERSEN, T. (1987b). The reflecting team: Dialogue and meta-dialogue in clinical work. *Family Process, 26,* 415–428.

ANDERSEN, T. (1991). *The reflecting team: Dialogues and dialogues about the dialogues.* New York: Norton.

ANDERSEN, T. (1992). Reflections on reflecting with families. In S. McNamee & K. J. Gergen (Eds.), *Therapy as social construction.* Newbury Park, CA: Sage.

ANDERSEN, T., & Naess, I. (1986). Four hearts and four families in dilemma. *Family Systems Medicine 4,* 96–106.

ANDERSON, H., & Goolishian, H. A. (1988). Human systems as linguistic systems: Preliminary and evolving ideas about the implications for clinical theory. *Family Process, 27,* 371–393.

ANDERSON, H., and GOOLISHIAN, H. (1992). The client as expert: A not-knowing approach to therapy. In S. McNamee & K. J. Gergen (Eds.), *Therapy as social construction.* Newbury Park, CA: Sage.

BAKHTIN, M. M. (1981). *The dialogic imagination.* Austin: University of Texas Press.

BALDESSARINI, R. J. (1990). Drugs and the treatment of psychiatric disorders. In A. G. Goodman, J. W. Rall, A. S. Nies, & P. Taylor (Eds.). *The pharmacological basis for therapeutics (8th ed.).* New York: Pergamon Press.

BANDLER, R., & GRINDER, J. (1982). *Reframing: Neuro-linguistic programming and the transformation of meaning.* Moab, UT: Real People Press.

BARLOW, C., EPSTON, D., MURPHY, M., O'FLAHERTY, L., & WEBSTER, L. (1987). In memory of Hatu (Hayden) Barlow (1973–1985). *Family Therapy Case Studies, 2,* 19–37.

BARSKY, A. (1988). *Worried sick: Our troubled quest for wellness.* Boston: Little, Brown.

BATESON, G. (1972). Conscious purpose versus nature. In G. Bateson (Ed.), *Steps to an ecology of mind.* New York: Ballantine Books.

BATESON, G., JACKSON, D., HALEY, J., and WEAKLAND, J. (1956). Toward a theory of schizophrenia. *Behavioral Science, 1,* 251–254.

BRATEN, S. (1987). Paradigms of autonomy: Dialogical or monological? In G. Geubner (Ed.), *Autopoiesis in law and society.* Hawthorne, NY: Walter de Gruyter.

BREUER, J., & FREUD, S. (1957). Fraulein Anna O. In J. Strachey (Ed.), *Studies on hysteria.* New York: Basic Books.

BRUNER, E. M. (1986a). Ethnography as narrative. In V. W. Turner & E. M. Bruner (Eds.) *The anthropology of experience.* Urbana: University of Illinois Press.

BRUNER, E. M. (1986b). Experience and its expressions. In V. W. Turner & E. M. Bruner (Eds.), *The anthropology of experience.* Urbana: University of Illinois Press.

BRUNER, E. M., & GORFAIN, P. (1984). Dialogic narration and the paradoxes of Masada. In E. M. Bruner (Ed.), *Text, play, and story.* Prospect Heights, IL: Waveland Press.

BUCHANAN, J. J., & OATES, W. J. (1957). *Boethius: The consolation of philosophy.* New York: Frederick Ungar.

CAMPBELL, T. (1986). *Family's impact on health: A critical review and annotated bibliography.* National Institute of Mental Health Series DN No. 6, DHHS Pub. No. (ADM)86-1461. Washington, DC: U.S. Government Printing Office. (Also available in *Family Systems Medicine, 4,* 135–328)

CHARNEY, D. S., WOODS, S. W., NAGY, L. M., SOUTHWICK, S. M., KRYSTAL, J. H., & HENINGER, G. R. (1990). Noradrenergic function in panic disorder. *Journal of Clinical Psychiatry, 51*(Suppl. A), 5–11.

CHASE, M. (1993). Version of PMS called disorder by psychiatrists. *The Wall Street Journal,* May 28, B1, B3.

CHIARI, G., & NUZZO, M. L. (1988). Embodied minds over interacting bodies: A constructivist perspective on the mind-body problem. *Irish Journal of Psychology, 9,* 91–100.

CLARK, C. R., GEFFEN, G. M., & GEFFEN, L. B. (1987). Catecholamines and attention II: Pharmacological studies in normal humans. *Neurosciences & Behavioral Reviews, 11,* 353–364.

COMMITTEE ON CHILDREN WITH DISABILITIES. (1987). Medication for children with an attention deficit disorder. *Pediatrics, 80,* 758–759.

CREED, F. (1989). Appendectomy. In G. W. Brown & T. O. Harris (Eds.), *Life events and illness.* New York: Guilford Press.

DAVID-MENARD, M. (1989). *Hysteria from Freud to Lacan: Body and language in psychoanalysis.* Ithaca, NY: Cornell University Press.

DE SHAZER, S. (1985). *Keys to solution in brief therapy.* New York: Norton.

DREYFUS, H. L., & WAKEFIELD, J. (1988). From depth psychology to breadth psychology: A phenomenological approach to psychopathology. In S. B. Messer, L. A. Sass, & R. L. Woolfolk (Eds.), *Hermeneutics and psychological theory: Interpretive perspectives on personality, psychotherapy, and psychopathology.* New Brunswick, NJ: Rutgers University Press.

ELMER-DEWITT, P. (1992). Depression: The growing role of drug therapies. *Time,* July 6, 57–60.

ENGEL, G. (1977). The need for a new medical model: A challenge for biomedicine. *Science, 196,* 129–136.

EPSTON, D. (1986a). Competition or co-operation? *Australian & New Zealand Journal of Family Therapy, 7,* 119–120.

EPSTON, D. (1986b). Night watching: An approach to night fears. *Dulwich Centre Newsletter* (Australia), 28–39.

EPSTON, D. (1992). "I am a bear": Discovering discoveries. In D. Epston & M. White (Eds.), *Experience, contradiction, narrative and imagination.* Adelaide, Australia: Dulwich Centre Publications.

EPSTON, D., & WHITE, M. (1992). *Experience, contradiction, narrative and imagination.* Adelaide, Australia: Dulwich Centre Publications.

FERNANDEZ, J. W. (1986). The argument of images and the experience of returning to the whole. In V. W. Turner & E. M. Bruner (Eds.), *The anthropology of experience.* Urbana: University of Illinois Press.

FISCH, R., WEAKLAND, J. H., & SEGAL, L. (1983). *The tactics of change: Doing therapy briefly.* San Francisco: Jossey-Bass.

FISHER, L., RANSOM, D. C., TERRY, H. E., & BURGE, S. (1992). IV. Family structure/organization and adult health. *Family Process, 31,* 399–419.

FIUMARA, G. C. (1990). *The other side of language: A philosophy of listening.* New York: Routledge, Chapman & Hall.

FLOR-HENRY, P. (1983). *Cerebral basis for psychopathology.* Boston: John Wright-PSG.

FORD, C. (1983). *The somatizing disorders: Illness as a way of life.* New York: Elsevier.

GADAMER, H.-G. (1976). *Philosophical hermeneutics.* Berkeley: University of California Press.

GALLAGHER, N. (1991). The revolution within. *The Family Therapy Networker,* March, 50–57, 78.

GEERTZ, C. (1986). Making experience, authoring lives. In V. W. Turner & E. M. Bruner (Eds.), *The anthropology of experience.* Urbana: University of Illinois Press.

GERGEN, K., & GERGEN, M. (1983). Narratives of the self. In T. R. Sarbin & K. E. Scheibe (Eds.), *Studies in social identify*. Westport, CT: Praeger.

GLENN, L. (1985). My face. In J. E. Sharpe (Ed.), *American Indian prayers and poetry*. Cherokee, NC: Cherokee Publications.

GOFFMAN, E. (1971). *Relations in public: Microstudies of the public order*. New York: Harper & Row.

GOLDMAN, C. R. (1988). Toward a definition of psychoeducation. *Hospital and Community Psychiatry, 39*, 666–668.

GOODWIN, D. W., & GUZE, S. B. (1984). *Psychiatric diagnosis* (3rd ed.). New York: Oxford University Press.

GOOLISHIAN, H. A., & WINDERMAN, L. (1988). Constructivism, autopoiesis and problem determined systems. *The Irish Journal of Psychology, 9*, 130–143.

GOTTLIEB, A. (1992). How to get people to do what you want. *McCall's, March*, 60–64, 151.

GRIFFITH, J. L., & GRIFFITH, M. E. (1992a). Owning one's epistemological stance in therapy. *Dulwich Centre Newsletter* (Australia), *1*, 11–20.

GRIFFITH, J. L., & GRIFFITH, M. E. (1992b). Speaking the unspeakable: Use of the reflecting position in therapies for somatic symptoms. *Family Systems Medicine, 10*, 41–51.

GRIFFITH, J. L., GRIFFITH, M. E., KREJMAS, N., MCLAIN, M., MITTAL, D., RAINS, J., & TINGLE, C. (1992). Reflecting team consultations and their impact upon family therapy for somatic symptoms as coded by Structural Analysis of Social Behavior. *Family Systems Medicine, 10*, 41–51.

GRIFFITH, J. L., GRIFFITH, M. E., MEYDRECH, E., GRANTHAM, D., & BEARDEN, S. (1991). A model for psychiatric consultation in systemic therapy. *Journal of Marital and Family Therapy, 17*, 291–294.

GRIFFITH, J. L., GRIFFITH, M. E., & SLOVIK, L. S. (1990). Mind-body problems in family therapy: Contrasting first- and second-order cybernetics approaches. *Family Process, 29*, 13–28.

GRIFFITH, M. E., & GRIFFITH, J. L. (1990). Can family therapy research have a human face? *Dulwich Centre Newsletter* (Australia), 2, 11–20.

HALEY, J. (1980). *Leaving home*. New York: McGraw-Hill.

HAMILTON, M. (1960). A rating scale for depression. *Journal of Neurology, Neurosurgery, and Psychiatry, 23*, 56–62.

HARTNACK, J. (1965). *Wittgenstein and modern philosophy* (2nd ed.). Notre Dame, IN: University of Notre Dame Press.

HEDERMAN, M. P., & KEARNEY, R. (1982). *The crane bag: Book of Irish studies*. Dublin: The Blackwater Press.

HEIDEGGER, M. (1949). *Existence and being*. Washington, DC: Henry Regnery.

HEIDEGGER, M. (1962). *Being and time*. New York: Harper & Row.

HEIDEGGER, M. (1971). *On the way to language*. New York: Harper & Row.

HERMAN, J. (1989). The need for a transitional model: A challenge for biopsychosocial medicine? *Family Systems Medicine, 7*, 106–111.

HOCHSCHILD, A. R. (1983). *The managed heart: Commercialization of human feeling.* Berkeley: University of California Press.

HOFFMAN, L. (1985). Toward a "second order" family systems therapy. *Family Systems Medicine, 3,* 381–396.

HOFFMAN, L. (1992). A reflexive stance for family therapy. In S. McNammee, & K. J. Gergen (Eds.), *Therapy as social construction.* Newbury Park, CA: Sage.

HOGARTY, G. E., ANDERSON, C. M., REISS, D. J., KORNBLITH, S. J., GREENWALD, D. P., JAVNA, C. N., & MADONIA, M. J. (1986). Family psychoeducation, social skills training, and maintenance chemotherapy in the aftercare treatment of schizophrenia. *Archives of General Psychiatry, 43,* 633–642.

HOLLISTER, L. E., & CSERNANSKY, J. G. (1990). *Clinical pharmacology of psychotherapeutic drugs* (3rd ed.). New York: Churchill Livingstone.

HOPPE, K. D., & BOGEN, J. E. (1977). Alexithymia in twelve commissurotomized patients. *Psychotherapy and Psychosomatics, 28,* 148–155.

HUBEL, D. H., & WIESEL, T. N. (1979). Brain mechanisms of vision. *Scientific American, 241,* 150–162.

JACOBS, B. L. (1986). Single unit activity of locus coeruleus neurons in behaving animals. *Progress in Neurobiology 27,* 183–194.

JACOBS, B. L. (1987). Central monoaminergic neurons: Single-unit studies in behaving animals. In H. Y. Meltzer (Ed.), *Psychopharmacology: The third generation of progress.* New York: Raven Press.

KANDEL, E. R. (1985). Nerve cells and behavior. In E. R. Kandel & J. H. Schwartz (Eds.), *Principles of neural science* (2nd ed.). New York: Elsevier.

KATZ, A., & DOYLE, G. (1986). A conversation with Tom Andersen. *The Society for Family Therapy and Research Newsletter, July–August,* 7–9.

KEARNEY, R. (1984). *Dialogues with contemporary continental thinkers.* New York: St. Martin's Press.

KELLY, G. A. (1963). *A theory of personality: The psychology of personal constructs.* New York: Norton.

KLEINMAN, A. (1977). Depression, somatization and the new cross-cultural psychiatry. *Social Science and Medicine 11,* 3–10.

KLEINMAN, A. (1983). Cultural meanings and social uses of illness behavior. *Journal of Family Practice, 6,* 539–545.

KLEINMAN, A. (1986). Some uses and misuses of the social sciences in medicine. In D. W. Fiske & R. A. Shweder (Eds.), *Metatheory in social science.* Chicago: University of Chicago Press.

KLEINMAN, A. (1988). *The illness narratives: Suffering, healing and the human condition.* New York: Basic Books.

KRAMER, P. D. (1993). *Listening to Prozac.* New York: Viking Books.

LIPCHIK, E. (1988). Interviewing with a constructive ear. *Dulwich Centre Newsletter* (Australia), *Winter,* 3–7.

MADANES, C. (1981). *Strategic family therapy.* San Francisco: Jossey-Bass.

MATURANA, H. (1988). Reality: The search for objectivity or the quest for a compelling argument. *The Irish Journal of Psychology, 9,* 25–82.

MATURANA, H. R., & VARELA, F. J. (1987). *The tree of knowledge: The biological roots of human understanding.* Boston: Shambhala.

MCCARTHY, I. C., & BYRNE, N. O. (1988). Mis-taken love: Conversations on the problem of incest in an Irish context. *Family Process, 27,* 181–199.

MCDANIEL, S., HEPWORTH, J., & DOHERTY, W. J. (1992). *Medical family therapy.* New York: Basic Books.

MENGEL, M. B., DAVIS, A. B., ABELL, T. D., BAKER, L. C., & RAMSEY, C. N. (1991). Association of family enmeshment with maternal blood pressure during pregnancy: Evidence for a neuroendocrine link explaining the association between family enmeshment and infant birth weight. *Family Systems Medicine, 9,* 3–17.

MERLEAU-PONTY, M. (1962). *Phenomenology of perception.* Atlantic Heights, NJ: Humanities Press.

MERLEAU-PONTY, M. (1964). *Sense and non-sense.* Evanston, IL: Northwestern University Press.

MERLEAU-PONTY, M. (1968). *The visible and the invisible.* Evanston, IL: Northwestern University Press.

MICHOTTE, A. (1963). *The perception of causality.* New York: Basic Books.

MINUCHIN, S., ROSMAN, B. L., & BAKER, L. (1978). *Psychosomatic families: Anorexia nervosa in context.* Cambridge: Harvard University Press.

MOORE, S. (1991). *Stanislavski revealed: An actor's guide to spontaneity on stage.* New York: Applause Theatre Books.

NIEUWENHUYS, R. (1985). *Chemoarchitecture of the brain.* New York: Springer-Verlag.

ORWELL, G. (1949). *1984.* New York: Harcourt Brace Jovanovich.

PALMER, R. E. (1969). *Hermeneutics.* Chicago: University of Chicago Press.

PAPP, P. (1983). *The process of change.* New York: Guilford Press.

PASK, G. (1976). *Conversation theory.* New York: Elsevier.

PELTO, P. J., & PELTO, G. H. (1978). *Anthropological research: The structure of inquiry* (2nd ed.). New York: Cambridge University Press.

PENN, P. (1982). Circular questioning. *Family Process, 21,* 267–280.

PENN, P. (1985). Feed-forward: Future questions, future map. *Family Process, 24,* 299–311.

POLKINGHORNE, D. E. (1988). *Narrative knowing and the human sciences.* Albany: State University of New York Press.

QVORTRUP, L. (1993). The controversy over the concept of information: An overview and a selected and annotated bibliography. *Cybernetics & Human Knowing, 1,* 3–24.

RANSOM, D. C., LOCKE, E., TERRY, H. E., & FISHER, L. (1992). V. Family problem-solving and adult health. *Family Process, 31,* 421–431.

ROBERTS, M., CAESAR, L., PERRYCLEAR, B., & PHILLIPS, D. (1989). Reflecting team consultations. *Journal of Strategic and Systemic Therapies, 8,* 38–46.

ROLLAND, J. (1990). Anticipatory loss: A family systems developmental framework. *Family Process, 29,* 229–244.

SAFFERMAN, A., LIEBERMAN, J. A., KANE, J. M., SZYMANSKI, S., & KINON, B. (1991). Update on the clinical efficacy and side-effects of clozapine. *Schizophrenia Bulletin, 17,* 247–161.

SARBIN, T. R. (1986). The narrative as a root metaphor for psychology. In T. R. Sarbin (Ed.), *Narrative psychology: The storied nature of human conduct.* Westport, CT: Praeger.

SELTZER, W. J. (1985a). Conversion disorder in childhood and adolescence. Part I: A familial/cultural approach. *Family Systems Medicine, 3,* 261–280.

SELTZER, W. J. (1985b). Conversion disorder in childhood and adolescence. Part II: Therapeutic issues. *Family Systems Medicine, 3,* 397–416.

SELVINI PALAZZOLI, M., BOSCOLO, L., CECCHIN, G., & PRATA, G. (1978). *Paradox and counterparadox.* New York: Jason Aronson.

SHORTER, E. (1992). *From paralysis to fatigue: A history of psychosomatic illness in the modern era.* New York: The Free Press.

SLOVIK, L. S., & GRIFFITH, J. L. (1992). The current face of family therapy. In J. S. Rutan (Ed.), *Psychotherapy for the 1990's.* New York: Guilford Press.

SLUZKI, C. (1990). Disappeared: Semantic and somatic effects of political repression in a family seeking therapy. *Family Process, 29,* 131–143.

SLUZKI, C., & RANSOM, D. (Eds.). (1976). *Double bind: The foundation of the communicational approach to the family.* New York: Grune & Stratton.

SMITH, G., MONSON, R., & RAY, D. (1986). Psychiatric consultation in somatization disorder. *New England Journal of Medicine, 314,* 1407–1413.

STEINER, G. (1989). *Martin Heidegger.* Chicago: University of Chicago Press.

TAYLOR, S. J., and BOGDAN, R. (1984). *Introduction to qualitative research methods* (2nd ed.). New York: Wiley.

TJERSLAND, O. A. (1990). From universe to multiverses—and back again. *Family Process, 29,* 385–397.

TOMM, K. (1987a). Interventive interviewing. Part I: Strategizing as a fourth guideline for the therapist. *Family Process, 26,* 3–13.

TOMM, K. (1987b). Interventive interviewing. Part II: Reflective questioning as a means to enable self-healing. *Family Process, 26,* 167–183.

TOMM, K. (1988). Interventive interviewing. Part III: Intending to ask lineal, circular, strategic, or reflective questions? *Family Process, 27,* 1–15.

TOMM, K. (1990, February). *Interventive interviewing.* Workshop presented for the 1990 Annual Conference of the Mississippi Association for Marriage and Family Therapy, Jackson, MS.

TUNKS, E., & BELLISSIMO, A. (1991). *Behavioral medicine: Concepts and procedures.* Elmsford, NY: Pergamon Press.

TURNER, V. W. (1986). Dewey, Dilthey, and drama: An essay in the anthropology of experience. In V. W. Turner & E. M. Bruner (Eds.), *The anthro-*

pology of experience. Urbana: University of Illinois Press.

U.S. COMMERCE DEPARTMENT. (1993). *1993 U.S. industrial outlook.* Washington, DC: U.S. Government Printing Office.

VARELA, F. J. (1979). *Principles of biological autonomy.* New York: Elsevier North-Holland.

VON GLASERFELD, E. (1988, June). *Discussant presentation in "Greek Kitchen in the Arctic."* Family Therapy Conference, Sulitjelma, Norway.

WALLIS, C., & WILLWERTH, J. (1992). Awakenings. Schizophrenia: A new drug brings patients back to life. *Time,* July 6, 52–57.

WHITE, M. (1986). Negative explanation, restraint, and double description: A template for family therapy. *Family Process, 25,* 169–184.

WHITE, M. (1988). The process of questioning: A therapy of literary merit? *Dulwich Centre Newsletter* (Australia), *Winter,* 8–14.

WHITE, M. (1989a). The externalizing of the problem and the re-authoring of lives and relationships. In M. White (Ed.), *Selected papers.* Adelaide, Australia: Dulwich Centre Publications.

WHITE, M. (1989b). Family therapy and schizophrenia: Addressing the "In the corner lifestyle." In M. White (Ed.), *Selected papers.* Adelaide, Australia: Dulwich Centre Publications.

WHITE, M. (1992). Deconstruction and therapy. In D. Epston & M. White (Eds.), *Experience, contradiction, narrative and imagination.* Adelaide, Australia: Dulwich Centre Publications.

WHITE, M., & EPSTON, D. (1990). *Narrative means to therapeutic ends.* New York: Norton.

WIENER, K., & KAGAN, J. (1976). Infants' reactions to changes in orientation of figure and frame. *Perception, 5,* 25–8.

WOOD, B., WATKINS, J. B., BOYLE, J. T., NOGUERIRA, J., ZIMAND, E., & CARROLL, L. (1989). The "psychosomatic family" model: An empirical and theoretical analysis. *Family Process, 28,* 399–417.

WRIGHT, L. M., & LEAHEY, M. (1987). *Families and chronic illness.* Springhouse, PA: Springhouse Corporation.

ZAMETKIN, A. J., NORDAHL, T. E., GROSS, M., KING, A. C., SEMPLE, W. E., RUMSEL, J., HAMBURGER, S., & COHEN, R. M. (1990). Cerebral glucose metabolism in adults with hyperactivity of childhood onset. *New England Journal of Medicine, 323,* 1361–1366.

Index